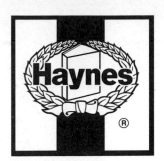

The Sex
Manual

Dr Ian Banks

Cartoons by Jim Campbell

(4086 - 152)

Models Covered
All genders, colours and orientations, age 16 and over

ABCDE
FGHIJ
KLMNO
PQRST
1 2 3

ISBN **1 84425 086 5**

British Library Cataloguing in Publication Data
A catalogue record for this book is available from the British Library.

Printed by **J H Haynes & Co Ltd,**
Sparkford, Yeovil, Somerset BA22 7JJ, England.

Haynes Publishing
Sparkford, Yeovil, Somerset BA22 7JJ, England

Haynes North America, Inc
861 Lawrence Drive, Newbury Park, California 91320, USA

Editions Haynes
4, Rue de l'Abreuvoir
92415 COURBEVOIE CEDEX, France

Haynes Publishing Nordiska AB
Box 1504, 751 45 UPPSALA, Sverige

Contents

Dedication
This book is dedicated to Hilary Martelli, sex goddess.

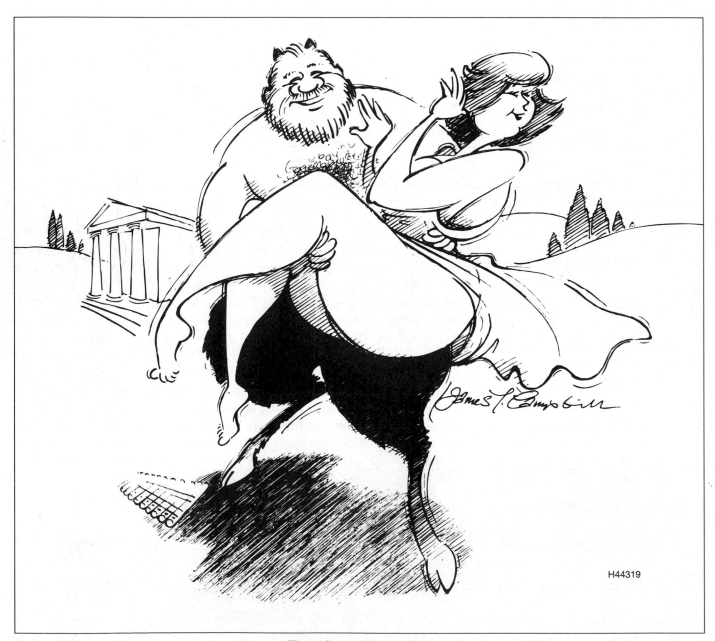

The author and his goddess

Sex is generally of the recreational variety. Just as well or there would be even more people around. Even so, it can be tiring, occasionally frustrating and often noisy. Putting this manual together was also fun but like sex itself more so when shared. A number of people who made sure the book was enjoyable, noisy and most of all safe need grateful acknowledgment from the author. Matthew Minter brought the book to a successful climax without losing breath while Jim Campbell was explicit in his interpretations of the written word. Simon Gregory was referred to for a second opinion. Special thanks to the people who wrote to me while working on the television set of The Good Sex Guide Late. I hope they can see themselves in this book and that their honesty and courage has not been betrayed. Presenters Toyah Willcox, Christine Weber and especially Suzi Hayman prevented premature exasperation.

The similarity between some sections of this book and NHS Direct On-Line are no coincidence. It is with grateful thanks we acknowledge the contribution of Bob Gann and the NHS Direct On-Line Healthcare Guide and Encyclopaedia.

Letters to the Author

All of these letters are genuine but have been altered slightly so as to protect the amazingly honest people who wrote them. You may see a bit of

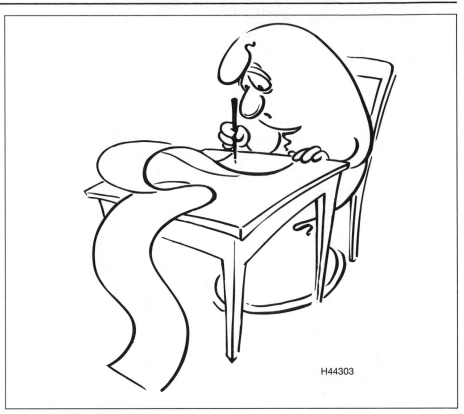

Dear Doctor...

yourself in these frank and sometimes sad letters. Thankfully some of them are hilarious; we are allowed to laugh at ourselves occasionally.

The Author and the Publisher have taken care to ensure that the advice given in this edition is current at the time of publication. The Reader is advised to read and understand the instructions and information material included with all medicines recommended, and to consider carefully the appropriateness of any treatments, practices and techniques mentioned. The Author and the Publisher will have no liability for adverse results, inappropriate or excessive use of the remedies, practices and techniques offered in this book or their level of effectiveness in individual cases. The Author and the Publisher do not intend that this book be used as a substitute for medical or other professional advice. In particular, advice from a medical practitioner should always be sought for any symptom or illness.

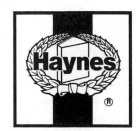

Sex is fun, but not entirely risk-free. These pages show just some of the potential risks and hazards, with the aim of creating a safety-conscious attitude.

General hazards

Burning

- Beware of friction burns from the carpet when having sex on the floor. Knee and elbow pads may provide some protection.

Fire

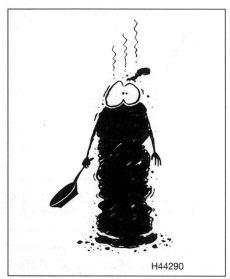

H44290

- Don't smoke in bed. Better yet, don't smoke at all.

- Be careful if using candles or incense to create a romantic atmosphere.

Intoxication

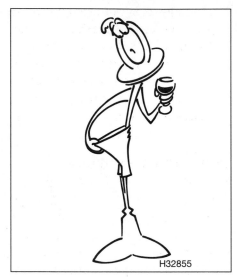

H32855

- Avoid consuming excessive amounts of alcohol before sex; it has an adverse effect on performance. Having sex with someone who is too drunk to give informed consent can lead to a charge of rape.

- Be aware of 'date rape' drugs such as Rohypnol and GHB. Don't leave your drink where other people can get at it. But don't be under any illusions – by far the commonest 'date rape' drug is alcohol.

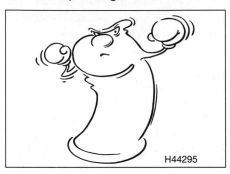

H44295

- People who are drunk are more likely to get into fights, especially if there is an element of sexual rivalry involved.

- Similar considerations apply to other recreational drugs.

Poisonous or irritant substances

- Keep them off your naughty bits – see *Allergies* in Chapter 6.

- If you've been handling chilli peppers, wash your hands thoroughly before handling anything else!

Older readers may remember the useful Mini van, complete with mattress in the back. A colleague who had struck lucky one night retired to the local beauty spot with his new lady friend. He dropped his trousers in the front seats while she was making herself comfortable in the back. The passion of the moment getting the better of him, he tipped the seats forward to give them the maximum amount of room and scrambled into the back as fast as

he could, slipping on to the floor as he did.

The resulting scraped knee didn't worry either of them and they got down to the matter at hand with the usual enthusiasm, until both became aware of an unfamiliar and increasingly unpleasant burning sensation 'down there'.

The same older readers will remember that the battery on a Mini van is located behind the driver's seat and

that the clamping arrangements are typically weak and ineffective. After a few years most Mini vans have their battery terminals completely exposed, the flimsy cover having been discarded long ago.

You know that white fluffy stuff that grows on the top of battery terminals? – especially those of older, knackered Mini vans? Well you really don't want to get any of that on your willy and so into your girlfriend...

Special hazards

Asphyxiation

- Some people derive pleasure from partial strangulation during sex. This is a most dangerous practice. Never put anything round your own or your partner's neck, or let anybody else do so to you.

- If you use a gag, it must not prevent mouth breathing.

Prosecution

- Rape is a criminal offence for which you can be imprisoned for a long time. It doesn't have to be violent – simply refusing to stop when the other party says 'no' can be rape.

- Having sex with someone below the legal age of consent, even if they agree to it, is also a criminal offence.

- Having sex in a public place is an offence, though you're unlikely to go to jail for it. Be discreet!

Sexually transmitted infections (STIs)

- Sexually transmitted infections are many and various – see Chapter 8. Condoms provide excellent protection against nearly all of them. *Always wear a condom when having penetrative sex.*

Unwanted pregnancy

- Another good reason for always using a condom. Do not rely on withdrawal (*coitus interruptus*), or so-called safe periods. And remember that the contraceptive pill does not protect against STIs.

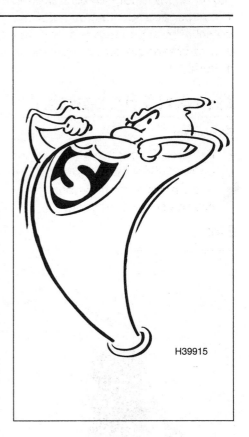

H39915

SAFER SEX

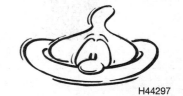

H44297

*When it comes to STIs, there's no such thing as totally safe sex – though you can eliminate about 99% of the risks by **always using a condom for any kind of penetrative sex**. The risk factors for the activities below are valid for most STIs.*

These activities are certainly high-risk	These activities are possibly risky	These activities are probably safe	These activities are certainly safe
Anal sex without a condom	Oral sex without a condom (on the penis) or other barrier (over the vagina or anus)	Anal or vaginal sex with a suitable condom	Cuddling, hugging, non-sexual massage
Vaginal sex without a condom	Sharing sex toys without sterilising them between users. (Or you can use condoms on a dildo)	Oral sex with a condom or other barrier	Kissing (without exchange of saliva)
Sharing drug injecting equipment	Sharing a toothbrush or a razor	Non-penetrative sex, including mutual masturbation	
		Kissing (with exchange of saliva)	

Chapter 1
Sex myths that just go on and on

Contents

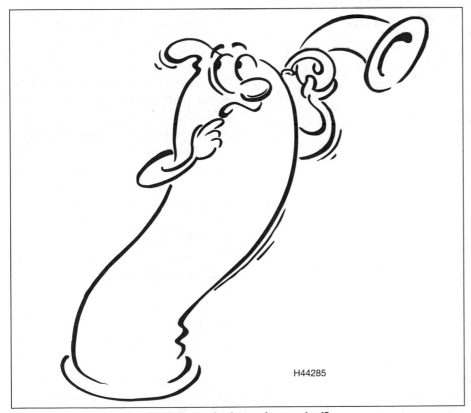

Does masturbation make you deaf?

1 Does masturbation make you deaf?

1 Given the horrendous hours junior doctors work, asking any casualty officer this question will invariably prompt a reply of 'Pardon?' In truth masturbation doesn't affect your hearing. Worse still it has no such effect on your mother's hearing either, who invariably rushed into your bedroom thinking you were being attacked by a Doberman with a stutter. Woody Allen knows a good thing when he experiences it. 'Don't knock it' he said in the film *Annie Hall*, 'it's sex with someone you love'. The Talmud states categorically, 'Thou shalt not masturbate either with hand or foot'. Yes, masturbation may not make you deaf but catching a genital verucca off your own foot really is the pits.

H44285

2 Is there something wrong with masturbating when you are having regular sex?

1 Masturbation is subtly different from sex. First it is almost one hundred per cent safe except when performed in zero gravity. Spacemen use the term Roger as a form of relief. Most men and women in stable, happy relationships also masturbate. This is where fantasy plays its part. Many people masturbate after sex to prolong the pleasure. This is particularly noted in couples where one or other of them falls fast asleep with the final gasp with little time to ask whether the earth moved for their partner also.

3 Can you get pregnant while you are breast-feeding?

1 This question is usually asked by the father of twelve children. Although there may be a prolonged delay in the resumption of periods, and thus ovulation, there is no way of knowing just when it is going to start. Obviously an egg has to be released for a period to follow. If unprotected intercourse takes place at this time there will be an even more prolonged delay. Getting pregnant is another excellent way of stopping periods.

4 Can you re-use a condom by turning it inside out?

1 Desperation is truly a terrible thing. The short answer to this question is yes, but your choice of sexual acquaintances may be severely restricted afterwards. You could also be a daddy as sperm can survive for a short space of time in the air. Additionally you may also contract just about any sexually transmitted disease going. But yes, you can re-use a condom by turning it inside out just like you can wear three day old socks by the same manoeuvre. On the other hand, it is probably best to shell out for another packet or have a cold shower. Both are a good deal cheaper in the long run.

5 Is petroleum jelly the best lubricant?

1 Yes, is the answer if you are talking about a baby's bum, but for use with a condom you would be wiser using sandpaper. At least you would feel the condom falling to pieces. Petroleum based lubricants will dissolve most condoms, particularly the ultra-thin varieties. As the bath towel puts it, 'Saying 'Oops' is not good enough'. Always use water-based lubricants; they are also a less of a fire risk during burning passion.

6 Is butter or margarine a good lubricant when using a condom?

1 No to both, even if you would never know it wasn't butter. Oil-based lubricants dissolve latex

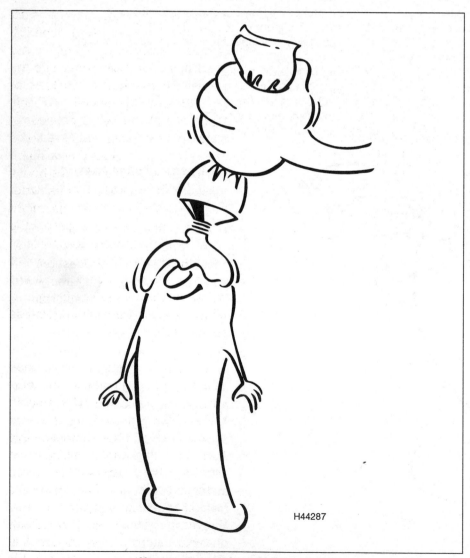

H44287

Always use water-based lubricants . . .

condoms – see above. Butter, margarine, cooking oil or even WD40 will produce a slippery slope towards a drippy willy not to mention unwanted fatherhood. Use only water-based lubricants.

7 Can you use a tampon to prevent pregnancy?

1 There is a doctor in England who uses tampons to stop severe nose bleeds. Walking around with a tampon up your nose has not yet hit the television advertisements. I suspect you might not feel quite so free if you walked into the local transport cafe in this nasally disadvantaged state. Tampons are a marvellous invention for soaking up blood such as the menses, or a nose bleed for that matter. Unfortunately they are not quite so good at stopping little genetic torpedoes hell bent on being the first successful headbanger. Not only will they not prevent pregnancy, they have even less protection against sexually transmitted diseases.

2 Part of a casualty officer's life is taken up by removing these machines after being rammed home in a fashion not unlike loading a cannon. Worse still they can be forgotten and fresh tampons used for the rest of the period. Removing them can then be hazardous as the tampon becomes saturated with offensive bugs a lot worse than headbangers. Septic shock is no joke and lives have been lost, so de-tampon before the fun with your ramrod, if you follow my drift.

8 If the man does not actually ejaculate can the woman get pregnant?

1 This is part of the, 'You can trust me, I'm in complete control' approach favoured by men who mistakenly put their money into the chewing-gum machine instead of the condom dispenser. As this fundamental error was caused by fifteen pints of lager you have some idea about just exactly how much control he will have over his bodily functions. If you like a bit of a flutter on the Grand National you might want to take your chance on the lager reaching those places three of sand and two of cement cannot reach. It will not, however, make any difference to your risk of picking up a nasty sexually transmitted disease such as HIV.

2 In terms of 'fates worse than death', men produce a pre-ejaculatory fluid designed to smooth the troubled waters for the following sperm. Even without ejaculation this fluid may contain sperm sitting in the pipeline from an earlier more successful mission. If any man asks you to accept this 'guarantee' you should first check whether he can chew the gum he bought and walk at the same time. Accepting his

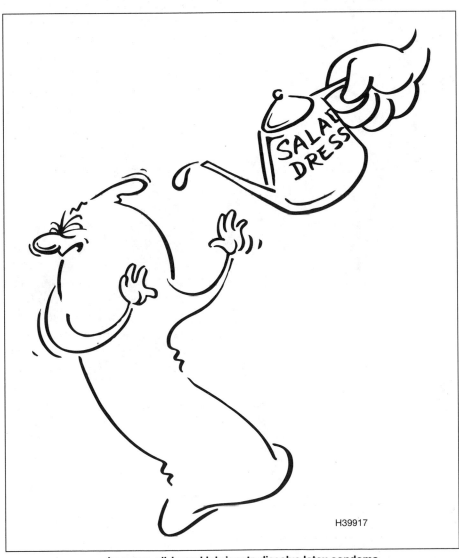

H39917

. . . **because oil-based lubricants dissolve latex condoms**

1

assurances entitles you to free chewing gum. Sit down while you eat as you might trip over your feet.

9 How long after sex can you take the morning after pill?

1 The so-called emergency contraceptive pill is simply a very high dose of sex hormones. It prevents a fertilised egg from implanting on the uterine wall. One dose is taken immediately followed 12 hours later by another. After 48 hours the chances of preventing pregnancy begin to decline. If left too long there is a theoretical danger of damaging the developing foetus without stopping the pregnancy. You will need a pregnancy test performed three weeks afterwards.

2 It is very effective but not in the same league as the oral contraceptive pill itself. You need a doctor's advice if you suffer from high blood pressure or have ever had a problem with blood clots.

10 Is cling film a suitable alternative to a condom in an emergency?

1 Obviously the word emergency means different things to different people. Cling film, or rubber gloves for that matter, are not a suitable alternative to anything except pockets full of tuna and cucumber, and smelly fingernails. Despite its name, cling film slips off very easily once wet. Similarly with rubber gloves unless you choose the fingers very carefully and with a fair degree of prescience. Worse still, phthalates present in plastic food wrappings may make the whole thing an academic exercise through chemical emasculation.

11 Does taking the Pill protect you from STIs?

1 STI stands for Sexually Transmitted Infection. The Pill most definitely does not stop you picking up fellow travellers. Condoms on the other hand will protect you from almost all nether region nasties *and* prevent unwanted pregnancies. Unfortunately men will often leave contraception all up to the woman.

Vaginal condoms are now available which really do protect a woman from a fate worse than death, in fact just death.

12 Can you can catch sexually transmitted diseases off a toilet seat?

1 This is the standard question from people who treat British bogs like some of those you find in French camp-sites. For the enlightenment of

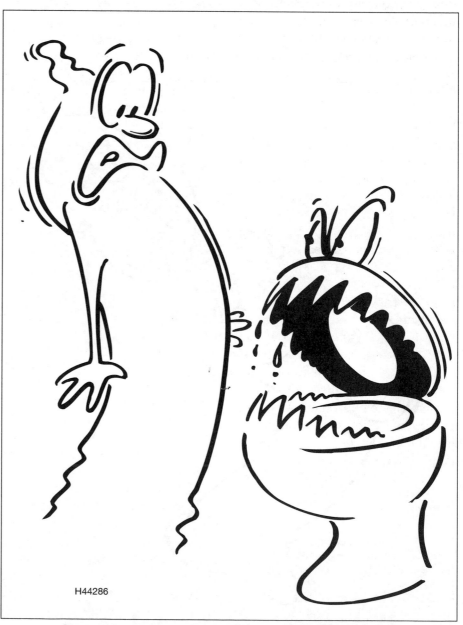

H44286

Can you can catch sexually transmitted diseases off a toilet seat?

those of you who always caravan instead, you stand over a small hole while attending to nature. This teaches you two things:

- If God was French he would have put eyes in our bums.

- French men prefer trousers without turn-ups.

2 On the plus side, your rear end never actually touches those parts that other people's rear ends have touched. At least not until you pull the chain and it flushes the entire loo area before you have a chance to get out of the door, slipping in the process.

3 Even so, sexually transmitted diseases are so called because that is how they are transmitted. Otherwise they would be called 'toilet transmitted diseases' and there would be no such things as turn-ups. Viruses such as the one which causes HIV cannot survive for any significant amount of time in the open air. Similarly bacteria and other small organisms responsible for these infections need body fluids to survive. This immunity does not extend to larger creepy crawlies like lice or crabs which can survive for a while, particularly their eggs which are laid on the pubic hairs. Mind you, telling your doctor that you picked up your itchy little hitch-hikers from a public loo may raise an eyebrow, but the treatment will be the same.

13 Can you only catch HIV if you are gay?

1 So far as scary myths go, this has to be the mother of them all. The virus which causes HIV is not politically correct. It has no preferences for any particular sex or the way they choose to make love. It is true that in the UK more gay than straight men have developed the disease but things are changing. We have a had a breathing space of a sort because the 'UK' virus strain is not as virulent as we first thought. There has not been the major epidemic once predicted. Enter a nasty variation on a theme. Some parts of the world have been devastated by the HIV virus, hitting men and women, gay and straight. Once this virus gets going in the UK there will be no second chances. Even with our present variety, unprotected casual sex, gay or straight, is near suicidal. A condom provides almost 100 per cent protection and beats the hell out of half a lemon. Some of them even taste better too, so I am told.

14 Can you get HIV from mouth to mouth resuscitation?

1 As most of the teenage population appear to be performing this life saving procedure on each other every Friday night, the answer is probably no. There is a theoretical risk from saliva which may contain infinitely tiny amounts of the virus, but this risk is so small as to be non existent. If the resuscitee is bleeding from the mouth this increases the risk but it is still relatively small. Blowing through a perforated piece of plastic barrier film further reduces the risk. At the end of the day you have to decide whether the small risk is worth it. The chances of meeting someone needing this attention who has HIV out of a population of 52 million is extremely small.

15 Is it possible to get stuck when making love?

1 Cramp is a dreadful invention. It always affects your calf just when you really don't want it to happen. Simply wiggling your little toe produces a pain equalled only by a meaningful relationship with Vlad the Impaler. Vaginismus is a cramp-like spasm which contracts the vagina. It is not so painful but it can be embarrassing. Some women even experience it when having a cervical smear performed. It can also occur during intercourse but the chances of endlessly doing the Lambada with your trapped partner round and round the kitchen are extremely small. More important is the discomfort it can cause for both of you. Extended foreplay, which does not mean asking, 'Are you awake Sheila?' can do the trick. That and a sense of humour along with a relaxed atmosphere. But not too relaxed, you don't want to fall asleep, Sheila.

16 Is it safe to have only one testicle?

1 This is a trick myth. Yes it is safe if you actually had the other one removed for whatever reason. An unremoved, undescended testicle increases your chances of cancer by at least four times. In terms of conferring immunity from becoming a father you are most definitely not safe. Each testis produces more than enough sperm to produce a chip off the old block. Similarly, your levels of testosterone will remain normal. The pituitary, a gland in the brain, controls the circulating amounts of sex hormone and simply prods the testicle into more action should levels fall.

1

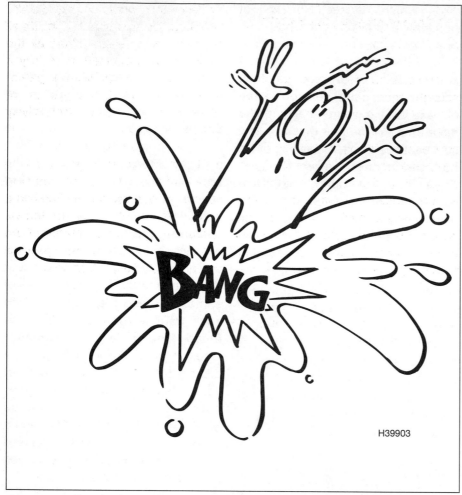

Does having sex on an aeroplane make your testicles blow up?

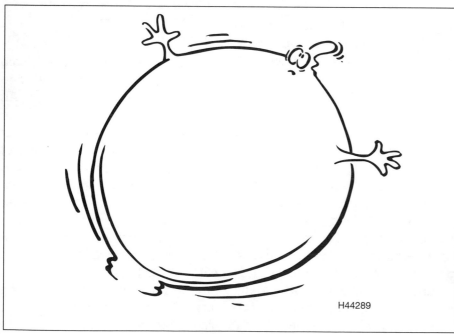

Can semen make you fat?

17 Does having sex on an aeroplane make your testicles blow up?

1 Fortunately not. Otherwise it would give terrorists a whole new dimension to plane hijacks. Members of the Mile High Club, an exclusive group of underweight individuals who loiter around airborne toilets, are particularly happy. 'You are aware of something which doesn't happen on the ground' one leading member who wishes to remain anonymous told me, 'perhaps it is the reduced cabin pressure'. More likely the cabin crew adjusting the video camera for the next office party. If you take a plastic mineral water bottle on board it will fizz far more on opening as the cabin pressure is maintained as the equivalent of that at a few thousand feet. This has no effect on the internal organs, or the external ones for that matter. Newton's law states, however, that to every action there is an equal and opposite reaction so you might like to tell your Mile High Partner to adopt the brace position.

18 Can semen make you fat?

1 Semen is a mixture of fructose (the same sugar as honey), an acid neutralising substance, minerals, lubrication fluid and tiny amounts of sperm. It has a calorific value similar to honey from very lazy bees. (Expert opinion varies – there's a surprise – but a figure of between 5 and 15 calories per average ejaculate seems to be the consensus.)

2 As far as oral sex is concerned,

then, whether the semen is swallowed or spat out doesn't really make much difference in terms of making the recipient fat. (There is a risk of passing on STIs though – see Chapter 8. If in doubt, use a condom.)

3 Absorption of semen in the vagina is poor and contributes little if anything in the way of energy. On the other hand the effort involved in getting it there is the equivalent of a five mile jog. On balance, therefore, semen definitely does not make you fat.

19 Can semen give you cancer?

1 There is no evidence that semen causes cancer. From an evolutionary point of view, it wouldn't really make much sense if all the females of a species promptly died a horrible death every time they tried to procreate. A sort of 'go forth and divide'. For many years a battle ranged over whether sex with uncircumcised men caused cervical cancer. It was noted that virgin women never contracted cervical cancer and that Jewish women in Israel had a lower incidence than women in, say, the UK. Obviously, the scientists thought, it's all down to the foreskin. When all the statistics are examined more fully it appears that promiscuity is a greater factor and that the presence or absence of the foreskin is of relatively little consequence.

2 It is worth noting that one organism suspected of causing cervical cancer is Human Papilloma Virus (HPV). This is transmitted by unprotected sex with a carrier of the virus; as ever, condoms provide more or less total protection.

1

Chapter 2
Kama Sutra

Contents

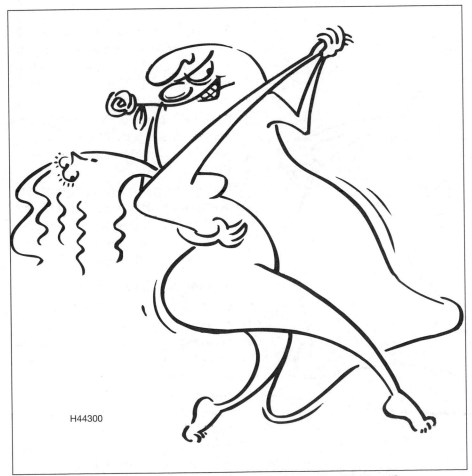

H44300

Who needs music when you both know the tunes off by heart?

1 Warming up: foreplay

1 One of the first casualties of a long term relationship is foreplay. Not surprisingly sex becomes indifferent and predictable once the prelude to sex is skipped. So OK, you might not be able to go through the whole gambit but there are other ways of keeping sex alive. Simply being aware of your partner's sexuality by commenting on the way they look, touching often, and allowing silences without the need to say anything other than with your eyes will keep that flame burning.

2 The home and particularly the bedroom naturally becomes the focal point for sex but foreplay can take place anywhere. When you are at a party or a meeting you can tell your partner a great deal about how you feel about them by simply catching their eye. A whisper in the ear along with an 'accidental' touch

2

somewhere naughty is part of the game of which there are only two players. This is not a reserve for teenagers, no matter how old you are, flirty behaviour, especially if 'illicit', is a real turn on. People having affairs talk of the sensuality of this kind of behaviour where the danger of being caught is part of the attraction. Restaurants are a great place for sending messages across a table, what happens underneath the table is your business, and keeping a straight face with your partner's toes wiggling in your groin while diners chomp away around you can be a real test of muscle control. Dancing is taken very seriously by the sex experts. It is your opportunity to talk to each other while moving closely together. You don't need to do it on a dance floor either and who needs music when you both know the tunes off by heart?

Gob smacked

3 Kissing is a very special form of foreplay even if it has been devalued by 'lovey' business people and PR types. Trying to work out how many times and which cheek to kiss first can lead to a comedy sketch worthy of Monty Python. A short peck of a kiss can set a million nerve fibres tingling. The lips and mouth have the greatest concentration of sensory nerves in the body. The big mistake though is to think only of lips-to-lips kissing. Try kissing the neck using your teeth as well, move up to the ears, biting the lobes gently, then move across the cheek to the lips, pressing them gently while letting your tongues seek each other out.

4 The other well-served parts of the body when it comes to sensation are the finger tips. Kissing them while stroking up and down sends a message of things to come which will not be lost on your partner and is significantly less embarrassing in polite company. It is a bit of a mystery why men have nipples but it is extremely fortunate when it comes to sex as they are every bit as sensitive as the female version and a kiss along with a nip of the teeth can make them rise to the occasion not to mention other, larger parts of the body.

5 People can be very aware of mouth odour and it can be a turn off. If you are drinking make sure both of you have the same taste! Most mouth odour comes from bad oral hygiene, not food. A tooth abscess can smell like a dead dog yet many people are completely oblivious to their own mouth odour. Breath fresheners only disguise the smell so see your dentist regularly if you really want kissing that stops your partner in their tracks rather than stun a skunk at a hundred paces.

Massaging the message

6 Most of us live under stressful conditions and find various ways of releasing the tension. Massage is one way of doing this, but it has a part to play in foreplay as well. You don't need to be an expert and the good news is that giving someone a massage can be as sexy as receiving one, remember the finger tips? Lying on a masseur's couch is not needed, simply coming up from behind your

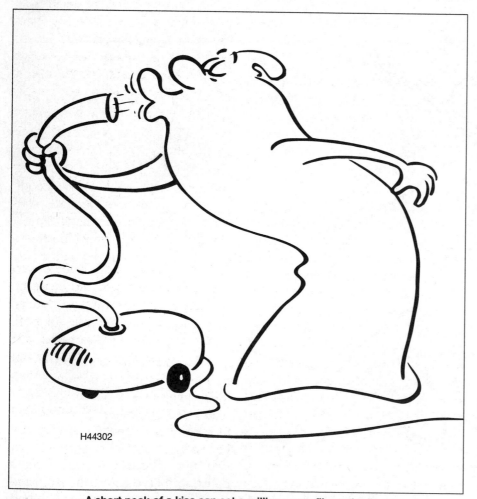

H44302

A short peck of a kiss can set a million nerve fibres tingling

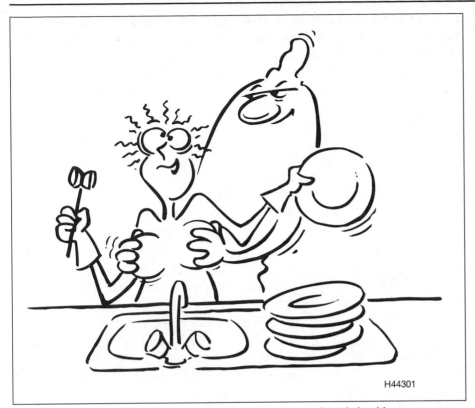

Simply coming up from behind will do the trick for a neck and shoulder massage

partner as they are sitting in a chair, working at the sink or even on the loo will do the trick for a neck and shoulder massage. For more elaborate jobs a scented oil enhances the pleasure as smell is the most basic and evolutionary primitive sense we possess. Don't overdo the scent though, the body's natural smell stimulates a very primitive part of the brain called the hippocampus and it will be masked by heavy-handed use of perfumes. And don't overdo the oil either if you're going to use a condom – remember that oil-based lubricants weaken condoms and can cause them to split.

7 Choose somewhere warm, cosy and (especially) where you will not be disturbed. Turn off the TV, radio, telephone, mobile phone and dog. A fluffy white towel is nice but not obligatory, but a firm base is a must. With a little oil use light touches all over their body while they lie on the face. You will sense where they are most tense in the way their muscles respond. Don't forget the sides of the body, stroking downwards towards the hips and buttocks. Use your thumbs, knuckles, flat of hand and finger tips. Now is the chance to explore the places of your partner's body you don't normally consider sexual, such as the soles of their feet, the inner thighs, the cleft of their buttocks. Don't go near the obvious places until you have aroused them fully with all the 'soft' areas. You will know when they desperately want you to massage the rising places. Don't rush, the fleeting, accidental touch will keep the suspense alive and make the final massage so much more satisfying. The final massage can involve a vibrator, a dildo, an empty cola bottle or the real thing. Your imagination is the only limit.

Oral sex

8 When it comes to foreplay, oral sex is probably the king and queen. It can be the climax of sex itself – knowing what you and your partner want is important. Penetrative sex is not always desired by one or both parties. Huge myths surround oral sex, but it is probably the safest form of sex and for some the most enjoyable. Whether it is really part of foreplay is debatable but it certainly gets your partner's attention. Crude attack can be part of the approach but subtlety often produces a better result all round. Dropping a fork or knife next to them at the dinner table and brushing your lips against their groin as you bend to retrieve the utensil can start the whole thing off. Don't rush with oral sex. Use your fingernails and lips on the inner thighs first, tiny 'accidental' kisses on the vagina or penis will stimulate more than a direct frontal attack. Knowing how sensitive your partner is does help; squeezing too hard on the testicles or biting the lips of the vagina too sharply will cause pain that will not translate into pleasure. Watch their faces for clues as you caress them. Remember that humour will surface so don't feel slighted if they giggle, join in.

9 It is up to you both whether you want penetrative sex. You might be perfectly satisfied having got this far. The name of the game is for both partners to enjoy and be comfortable with sex between you. Climax is not always required, a closer loving embrace is just as important in the long run, and it can be a pretty long run at that.

For him

10 Despite the name blow job, suck don't blow. Better still, lick or hold

2

his testicles in your mouth while stroking his penis, then take his penis into your mouth. You don't need to take it all, you can judge for yourself. For some women ejaculation into their mouths is extremely exciting, for others it is a turn off. Settle this with your partner first as one or both of you could be disappointed. A variation is to let him come over your breasts. It is your body, you decide.

For her

11 Women are even more keen on the gentle subtle approach than are men. Licking the thighs while playing with the lips of the vagina, caressing the clitoris and gripping the buttocks all add to the suspense. Using a finger first, press into her vagina, use your tongue at the same time then just your tongue and lips. Her clitoris may get larger and there will be a dampness, she may even wee as she gets excited. Consider this a compliment. Carrying on is a real turn on for many women. Don't be afraid to use a dildo or vibrator.

12 Note that although men often come quite quickly during oral sex, it may take a lot longer for the woman to come – some studies suggest around 20 minutes.

2 Positions

1 American police use a command, 'adopt the position'. Unless you have seen plenty of cop vs. bad guy movies this could lead to dangerous confusion. Sex is a bit like that, according to ancient Indian and Oriental texts there are at least 1000 positions. The Kama Sutra is not quite so informative but still has a baffling number of variations on the basic theme, none of which require wardrobes, for the jumping off. Like the Arabian Nights stories, you could take a very long time getting through all of these. The latest estimate of average sexual frequency in the UK is once per week, which means it will be around 20 years if you want to sample them all before you get back to the first position. As some of them require the muscular flexibility of Houdini you might want to go for them first before the arthritis sets in. Imagination and a sense of humour are vital assets, as are various bits of furniture.

69

The number says it all really. Simultaneous oral stimulation is popular and there are many variations on the theme. For some people it is too distracting but for many it is the ultimate foreplay. Try placing pillows under the head and hips of the 'below' partner. Remember there are more areas to touch and play with than the vagina or penis. The thighs are very sensitive, particularly close to the penis or vagina. It can also tickle so expect some uncontrollable chuckles. The anus is badly neglected by most couples for fear of 'perversion' or being unhygienic. Generally speaking oral sex is sadly lacking in surgical cleanliness so a furtive massage and kiss around the buttocks will not make so much difference. Tonsils are useful for many things but are not happy with large hot penises slapping them around the head and neck. The woman can control her partner's oral penetration by judiciously squeezing his buttocks or pressing on his hips. If this sounds too energetic, go for the Golden Spoon. Lie head to tail on your sides with one leg bent and raised. With your head on your partner's inner thigh, gently use your mouth and tongue to reach those places many lagers fail to reach. Nice way to fall asleep.

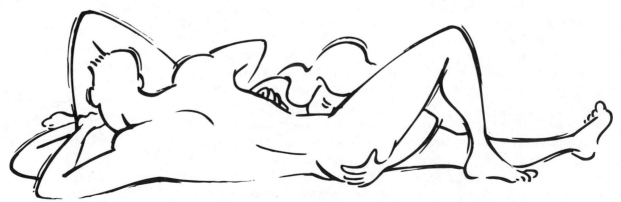

69: Simultaneous oral stimulation

H44308

Men with a mission

Along with beads and bibles the early Christian missionaries preached 'godly sex' to their converts. Other than face-to-face with the man on top there was only 'godless sex'. This says a great deal about male domination and the perceived value of procreation vs. fun. Even so, it does provide great pleasure, especially if the woman raises her hips (a pillow can help) and the man uses his pubic bone to rub against the clitoris. This is where the missionary position and fun part company. Use your hands to explore those bits some missionaries can't reach. Gently playing with the testicles, breasts, anus and vagina can make an orgasm truly explosive.

Missionaries on their knees

One definition of a gentleman is he who takes most of his weight on his elbows. The kneeling position can give better penetration without that crushing feeling. This is a big advantage if either of you is a tad overweight. Even better if you use a bed or low settee for her to lie on. Can be sore on the knees though so choose somewhere soft like a rug if you are going for the marathon. Housemaid's knee is a rare complication of sex, but why tempt fate?

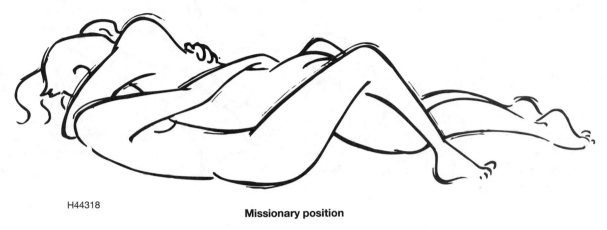

H44318

Missionary position

Emperor rules OK

Thai concubines were discussing positions before the UK was coming to terms with which particular woad to wear on posh occasions. The Emperor got its name from its element of male control, as the man is higher and is calling the shots. He kneels back on his heels, pulling the reclining woman towards him with her knees pulled to her shoulders. Watching the meeting of penis and vagina is a real turn on for both, especially if she likes the feeling of surrender. Lifting her hips to change the angle of penetration along with thrusting deeper only serves to enhance this feeling. Feet usually get in the way while dancing but now they have a life of their own by stroking the man's lips, breasts and arms.

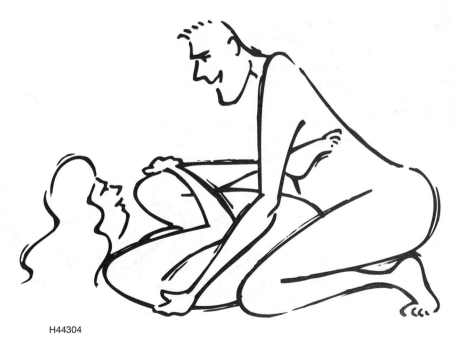

H44304

Emperor

2

Lovers' Knot

Lovers' Knot is a position not unlike the Emperor, but is a little more exacting for the woman as she needs fairly supple hips. Starting off in the Emperor position, the woman places her feet against the man's chest while she locks her arms around his waist. This way she can turn and twist her vagina against his penis. It can help if you were a boy scout but chanting 'we're riding along on the crest of a wave' never goes down well, even over a camp fire if I remember rightly.

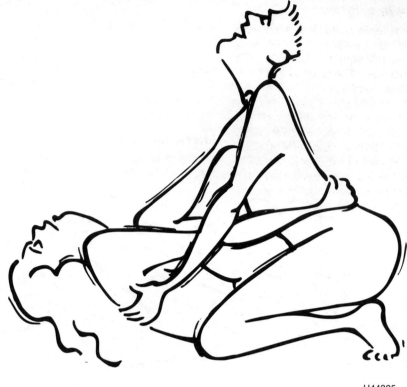

Lovers' Knot

H44305

Moon is a balloon

Catching the Moon is another variation where the woman gains control, a sort of Empress rather than Emperor. The man is still on top, but the woman holds his penis as he leans forwards with his legs stretched out in front of him. She bends her legs over his thighs. She is now in control as he can move his hips only slightly. Where this name comes from is anyone's guess but given the dexterity required it probably only happens once a month.

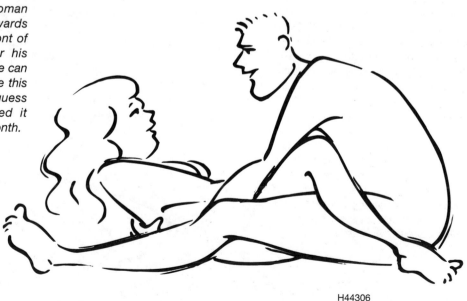

H44306

Catching the Moon

Cane pain

The Kama Sutra has a lot to answer for when it comes to mixing pain with pleasure. Splitting the Bamboo is a good example. The woman lies back with pillows under her hips while the man sits between her thighs. She now bends a knee and the man holds her foot by the ankle while her other foot is hooked over his opposite shoulder. Gently, he now moves her leg from his shoulder to the floor and back again. Imagine trying to take off a chicken leg. On second thoughts don't.

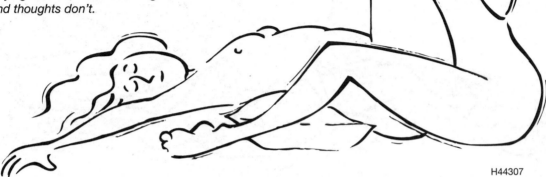

H44307

Splitting the Bamboo

Goose and ganders

Shakti is the antithesis of the missionary position and named after the Hindu goddess. On both counts early Christian missionaries will be turning in their urns. Best of both worlds, the woman is in charge while the man can lie back and relax with a good view. Many women favour this position because it allows them to press the penis against the G spot on the front wall of the vagina. It's not all squelch either, you can kiss and caress each other's hairy bits and breasts. Depending on his muscles or her shoe size he can lift the woman up and down on his penis. Great for the pecs and abs guys, and beats the hell out of crunches in the gym.

Shears for tears

While there are an apparently unlimited number of variations on the Shakti theme, a popular (if potentially painful) one is the Shears position. Get yourself into the classic Shakti position, then let the woman lie backwards until her head is between the man's ankles. OK, not for those with a fear of fractured penises, but it does force the penis against the woman's G spot and allows the man to play with her clitoris at the same time. Great chance to check for verrucas as well.

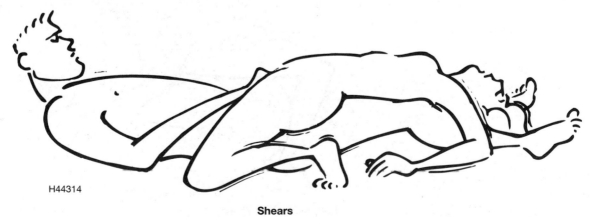

H44314

Shears

2

Papillon

Keeping one knee on the floor or bed and the other stretched out like a runner at the blocks, the woman then draws her partner up to her with a hand under his lower back while turning her hips and thrusting her pelvis. Lying backwards on his chest gives him the chance to caress her breasts and vagina. This is known as the Butterfly. Steve McQueen and Dustin Hoffman never even thought about it, but then they had other things on their mind.

H44315

The Butterfly

Hot pants on a hot seat

This is the ultimate fantasy for a woman who likes to pass water while making love. The man lies on his back with his legs drawn to his chest. She then sits on top of his penis and buttocks. She can now hold his testicles while he supports her waist. Golden Showers all round folks, don't forget to change the sheets.

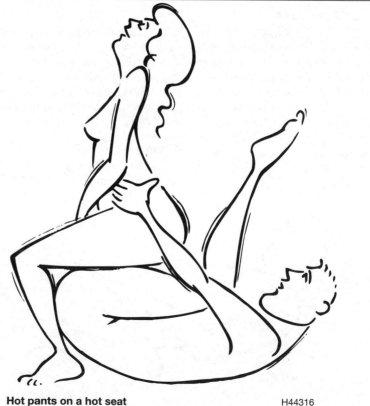

Hot pants on a hot seat

H44316

Horse riding

Imagine a horse with a penis on its back. Or a surf board with the same accessory. Now you have the idea. The man lies on his back with the woman astride on his penis. She is in control and can rock backwards and forwards. For him he can lie back and enjoy. The surf's up, as they say.

H39926

Horse riding

Monkey business

Like whales, monkeys have sex in lots of different ways including gay sex. Not weighing 24 tons is an advantage for having sex in trees, along with not having a hole in the top of their heads. People are not much different either, if you exclude tails and using bananas for more than simply eating. Sitting back on his ankles with the woman between his legs gives a pretty good approximation to the favourite monkey position. Holding on to the end of the bed gives a bit of leverage too. Monkeys use this as an opportunity to groom their partner and pick out any fleas or ticks. Being naked apes has a certain advantage.

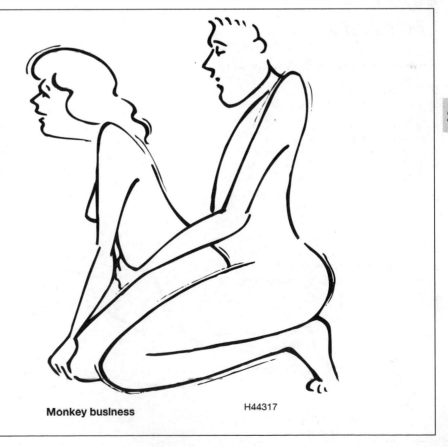

Monkey business

H44317

2

Woof woof love

The doggie is popular not least because it is relatively gentle, allowing you both to be less athletic but providing deep penetration. While on all fours the woman is entered from behind. This is an opportunity to try anal sex which is now legal between consenting UK adults of whatever sexual combination. Be gentle and use plenty of lubrication. Whichever route chosen, you can stimulate each other by playing with the testicles and vagina/breasts.

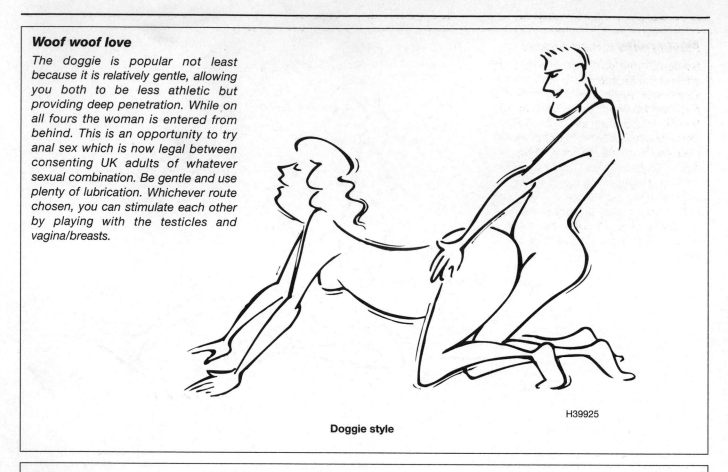

H39925

Doggie style

Feline fun

Any position with a name like the Piercing Tiger can't be all bad. Named in ancient Hindu, it is also known as the Sphinx. You can get some idea of the position by thinking of the way big cats mate. The male leaps on the back of the female and bites her neck to hold her down (and prevent getting eaten like the praying mantis). The human variety involves the woman lying on her face with legs open or apart. The man lies on top face down. It is a real fantasy trip as the male is all dominant and the woman cannot see what he is doing. The Sphinx bit kicks in as the woman rests her elbows in front of her. Hopefully there will not be too much sand about.

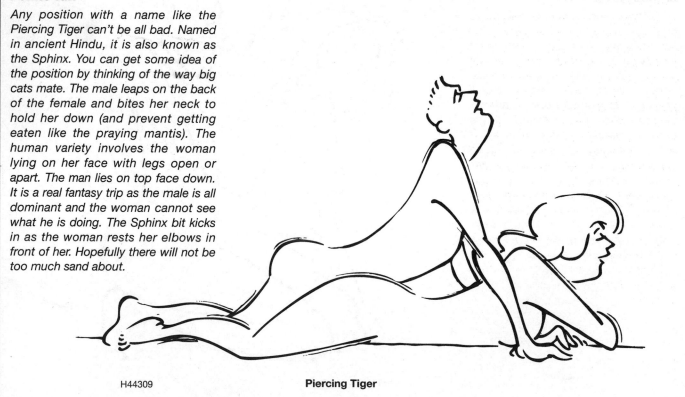

H44309   **Piercing Tiger**

Playing with forked tongue

Serpents feature prominently in ancient texts and were considered very power magic. They also mate in a peculiar manner, described in the human variation as the Folded Serpent. Basically the woman bends over and touches her toes, holds her ankles or holds the man's ankles between her legs. The man enters from behind. Make sure there is something soft to fall on to as balance is a tad on the tricky side. People with slipped discs might want to give this one a miss.

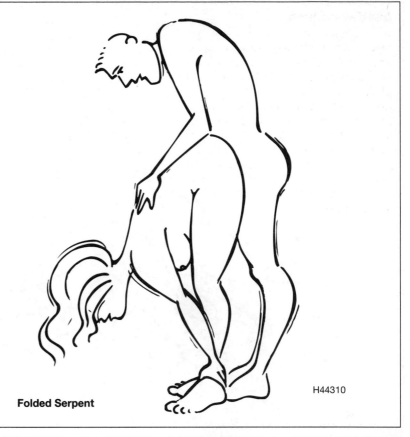

Folded Serpent

H44310

Veggie sex

Its not just animals that can teach us about positions, plants can show us a thing or two as well. Sadly, there is no mention of the Venus Fly Trap in the ancient texts. Vines do pop up in various places, showing the importance attached to them and to wine for that matter. If there is an aphrodisiac it has to be a single glass of fine red wine. After ten glasses it also doubles up as an excellent form of family planning. The Climbing Vine position is not for the faint-hearted and requires some muscle power on the man's side. This overcomes differences in height which can make standing sex ('a knee-trembler') more difficult. The man lifts the woman onto his penis and she remains in place by wrapping her legs around his hips. This can be helped by using an overhead bar or rope. Not to be attempted after the 10th glass of wine, or the 6th for that matter.

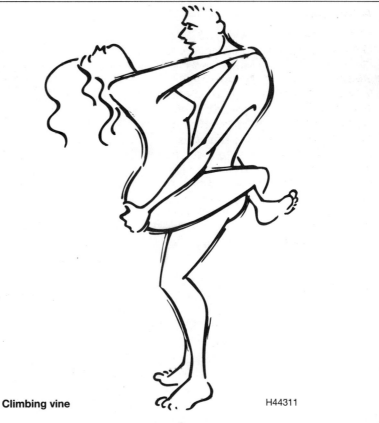

Climbing vine

H44311

2

A weight off your mind

If either of you is overweight or the woman is pregnant you might want to think about side-to-side love making. It can also be a lovely way of dropping off to sleep together. Face-to-face is more difficult than from the rear but even so by lifting one leg over the man's hips the woman can be brought much closer. The Cradle is a variation which allows face-to-face contact but is less tiring than the missionary position. Pregnant women particularly like this position as it give them better control despite the 'bump'. She lies on her back lowering her legs over the man's hips as he lies on his side facing her. She can keep her legs together as he enters which makes it more stimulating.

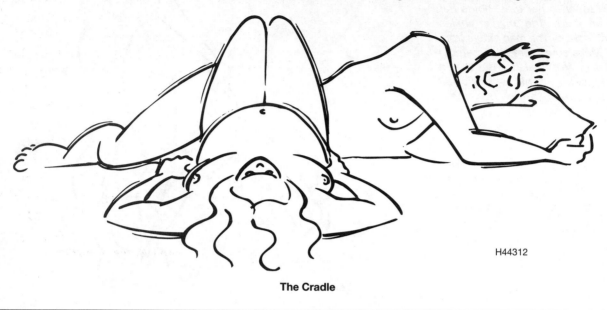

H44312

The Cradle

Spoonerisms

Perhaps the most gentle and least tiring position is that of Spoons. This is ideal for tired couples who need their sleep but want a loving goodnight send off to dreamland. Lying on their sides the man enters from behind with his body following the contours of the woman. Again, this is very useful if she is pregnant. It also gives the opportunity to caress breasts, face, tummy and vagina. Handy if one or other has been eating garlic too.

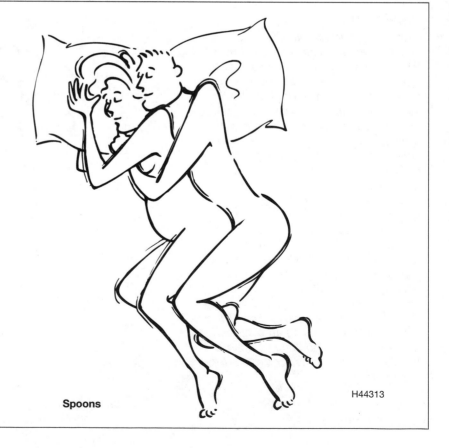

Spoons

H44313

Dear Doctor

At the age of 52 I had my first sexual experience which only lasted a few weeks, but now I am living with my first proper partner. The only problems we have are sexual and there's not much fun at all in the bedroom, which is mostly because he is so much taller, heavier (18 stone), stronger and more experienced than me. I try to please him but he says he is master of the bedroom and doesn't understand that I am frightened of his weight falling on top of me. He rests his hand on my right shoulder to support himself, but it's arthritic and hurts plus I worry his hand is going to slip and go round my throat. This means I am always tense and just want to get sex over with. Frequently our love making ends in frustration with him shouting and me trying not to cry which drives him mad. I don't like going on top of him because I've put on lots of weight since I met him. He's such lovely man in every other way and when sex is good, it's wonderful. I don't want to lose him but it's making me very stressed out and I can't sleep well. Please help.

Communication between lovers is not always the best. Your partner's dominance is only acceptable if it is acceptable to you. He can still feel the dominant partner without scaring you half to death but you do need to talk about it to him. Putting on weight is paradoxically a sure sign of being unhappy over something. Eating makes you feel better and able to cope. Unfortunately over-eating only makes things worse which then makes you eat even more. A vicious circle. You could experiment with different positions such as him behind with you on your side. Once the element of fear is removed you should be able to enjoy sex again and this will help both of you. At the end of the day you are going to think about your future and (if things do not improve) whether you can live with the fear.

3 Sex during pregnancy

1 Although the myth and mystery is being taken out of pregnancy to the extent that even men are beginning to understand it, there is still fear that sex is taboo. Strict rules used to be enforced over sex during pregnancy, but as the baby is virtually immune from harm during love making, sex is safe at all stages of pregnancy, right up to the date the baby is due. A too liberal interpretation of this general observation can provide no end of entertainment for the labour ward staff.

2 There are some important exceptions requiring caution and possibly abstinence from penetrative

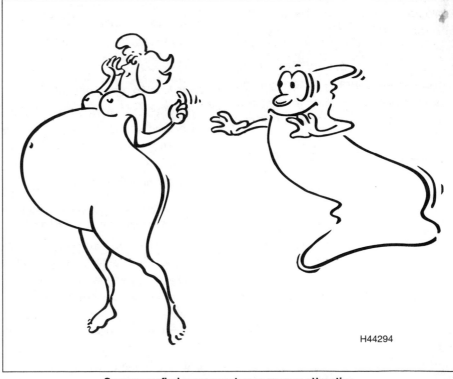

H44294

Some men find a pregnant woman very attractive

sex. If in doubt you should seek the advice of your obstetrician.

- If there have been repeated miscarriages.

- A series of premature labours.

- Placenta praevia (where the placenta lies close to or over the opening of the womb).

- If there is any bleeding during intercourse.

- If the waters have already broken.

3   In late pregnancy, because of the growing foetus, women may find the 'man on top' position uncomfortable and be more relaxed, happy and comfortable if you try the side-by-side or rear-entry positions. Many women are more comfortable when they lie on top.

Sexual desire

4   Male attitudes vary towards the appearance of their partner as pregnancy changes her shape. Some men find it very attractive, while others confess, often guiltily, that they find it a big turn-off. However, the phenomenon cannot be ignored. There is no rule that says you must find your pregnant partner attractive and equally you are not a pervert if it makes the hormones race.

5   During pregnancy, changes in a woman's sexual desire and in her sexual responses are usual. Some pregnant women have a reduced sexual interest in the first half of pregnancy, which continues, with considerable individual variation, through the second half of pregnancy. Reduced sexual

appetite can be misinterpreted as rejection.

6   There are of course other ways of showing and making love than penetrative sex. It is always best to talk about this as you can often find ways of helping each other. Spending a longer time in body contact with each other, without being demanding, will help maintain confidence in your relationship.

Myths

Penetrative, vaginal sex causes an abortion

- Untrue. The penis cannot enter the womb. Your doctor will advise you if there are any good medical reasons not to have sex.

Sex can damage the baby

- Untrue. The baby is well out of harm's way during intercourse. It is possible to introduce sexually transmitted diseases such as HIV which could affect your partner and possibly your baby, but you can be tested for these complaints. Meanwhile, use condoms, male or female.

Sex can lead to premature labour

- There is no evidence for this, although there are some conditions in which caution should be exercised. Again, your doctor will advise you.

An orgasm when pregnant will injure the baby or start labour prematurely

- Untrue. An orgasm can bring on contractions which are normally present towards the end of pregnancy called 'Braxton Hicks' contractions. They will settle on their own in a short time. Previous premature labours may require caution and your doctor will advise you.

Normal part of life

7   It is always worth remembering, not least because some doctors can forget, that pregnancy is not the same as being sick. Pregnant women are not 'patients'. Most women are more healthy during pregnancy than at any other time in their lives. Pregnancy is a normal part of life and is remarkable for the lack of problems that actually occur.

8   Having a baby can take its toll on the body. Many of the changes are temporary and can be reversed with some simple exercises and diet.

9   Stretch marks are areas of altered skin. Collagen maintains skin elasticity. This is reduced with ageing or by scarring. The skin loses its normal pigmentation. They are more noticeable if the woman is overweight, so losing some pounds will make them smaller, like the writing on a balloon when it deflates. Creams containing Vitamin E and A derivatives are said to help return skin back to its normal condition.

10 Some women find their vagina is too loose after having a baby. Passing something the size of a rugby ball and twice as hard through the pelvis is bound to have some effect on the vagina. If this is a major problem it can be solved with relatively simple surgery.

11 Episiotomy (cutting the perineum to avoid tearing during birth) is controversial and avoided whenever possible. The repair can be remarkably good at restoring normal service, but some women still find sex uncomfortable afterwards. These repairs used to be performed by the most junior doctors or even medical students. Now only senior

staff and highly trained midwives, under supervision if necessary, are allowed to put together those parts no man should let asunder.

12 Some women suffer from vaginal dryness for a while after giving birth. This can cause a vicious circle of anxiety, with dryness leading to pain and round again to anxiety over the next attempt at making love. Foreplay and relaxation are essential. Use a lubricant if necessary.

4 From the bottom up

1 Anal sex is now legal in the UK between consenting heterosexual adults. It was previously made legal for consenting gay men and the law has been brought into line. Despite changes and fluctuations in laws all over the world, people have been practising anal sex for countless generations and it is well described in the literature. Similarly, warnings of dreadful things which befall people who indulge in this form of sexual play have not yet brought the human race to its knees, a popular position in the first place. Paradoxically it is used as a form of birth control in many cultures, which may explain its abhorrence to some religions.

2 More liberated experts are quite happy when it comes to anal sex in homosexual relationships, as if gay men somehow are gifted with extra durable anuses. Common sense dictates that it is safe so long as simple hygiene and safer sex are

Dear Doctor

I have lived with my boyfriend for 18 months and we have a very good sex life. However, because of the publicity given to anal sex, he now wants us to try it and I thought I would write to you for your advice. I can see that from a man's point of view anal sex is probably not very different from vaginal sex except that perhaps the anus may be a tighter fit and more pleasurable. But I would like to know what sexual satisfaction I will get? For example, can I have an orgasm? Also, should he use a condom?

Trying to describe what anal sex is like to someone who has never experienced it is rather like explaining what it is like in a maze to someone with a similar lack of experience. It is impossible to issue a realistic answer as you may find the experience unpleasant, painful and/or humiliating. On the other hand it may be one of the most sexually exciting experiences you have ever had. Judging from its popularity within the gay community there is unlikely to be any danger. You should however, practise safer sex and using a condom makes good sense anyway because it can prevent the transmission of bacteria from the anus to your vagina. Use plenty of lubricant and the eternal phrase 'be gentle with me'.

employed. Without putting too fine a point on it, the anus is full of things you would not want on your cornflakes. At the same time, oral sex involves some pretty intimate contact with places not a million miles away.

3 It's a safe bet that the anus was not designed by evolution for sex. But then few people get pregnant by oral sex either. If you like it, and not all of us do, then fine. Use plenty of lubricant and proceed gently. Keeping clean, and using safer sex, makes sense for all modes of entry, as it were.

Dear Doctor

My wife and I practise anal sex a lot and we both really enjoy it. However, am I really being fair to her to want sex in this way all the time? We always use a condom and so all I'm really doing is checking if what we are doing is OK and won't do any harm.

Anal sex has been around for as long as, er, anuses. It is favoured by some groups as a form of contraception and during menstruation. Gay men practice anal sex with relatively little physical harm so long as safer sex is practised. If your partner is happy with the relationship, then fine but I do suspect that she would like some vaginal sex if only to relieve the boredom. You are using an organ which gives you great pleasure while she is not using hers. The simple answer is to ask her without applying pressure one way or the other, if you will excuse my turn of phrase.

2

5 Carma Sutra

1 Sorry about the pun, we couldn't resist it. The association between sex and cars goes back a long way. (Freud thought that women were aroused by cars because of the symbolism of pistons moving in and out of cylinders, but the American writer James Thurber pointed out that this was unlikely to be true, at least for the females in his family, because none of them had the slightest idea of how the internal combustion engine worked.) Here, then, are a few stories and suggestions for positions particularly suitable for use in, on or around cars. Not all of them will suit everybody – it depends on the size and agility of you and your partner, and of course on the size of the car.

2 Depending on who owns the car, what the upholstery is made of and what you expect to be doing, it may be a good idea to spread out a towel or blanket before you start.

3 Remember that having sex in public is illegal in the UK. Even if you don't reckon there's much risk of being arrested, you should not cause offence to innocent passers-by. But mind you don't get stuck while seeking seclusion!

4 Some of the positions show one partner or the other holding on to the steering wheel. This is only for support. Having sex while driving is both illegal and potentially dangerous.

My girlfriend and I used to go 'green-lane-ing' for some private in-car entertainment. One time we took the privacy aspect a little far and drove way too far down a lane, such that there was barely enough room either side to open the doors much more than a sliver. The trouble started when it came to going home time. Reversing in the dark with steamed-up windows is tricky at the best of times, but for a new driver, with banks on both sides and a dodgy battery to restart a cold, stalled engine? Not recommended. We had to clamber out the side with most space and walk to a friend's house and brazen it out while asking for a tow. Of course, the car started first time, and he reversed it straight out, which added to the embarrassment factor (along with the fact that my 'current' was his 'ex').

The Mini is quite a challenge but if clothes pegs are used to clip onto the seat covers, holding the seats in the 'up' position, then a couple who are small in stature may indulge in a limited repertoire. Missionary is the obvious but not exactly adventurous option, but variations of 'doggie' are far more interesting & entertaining. May I recommend a good yoga class?

I can confirm that the VW Jetta affords the would-be couple intent on love making plenty of space. The back of the front passenger seat folds right down to an almost horizontal position, allowing the man full access for anything he has in mind.

One warning to those people who have a glass sunroof. If one of you wants to put your feet up, be careful not to leave footprints on the glass. Otherwise you may find a son or daughter looking up and saying "look mummy someone has been walking on our roof in their bare feet and they have left their footprints behind."

Hint for motorcyclists – if the urge comes upon you and your beloved so strongly that you feel inclined to pull over straight away, but the ground's too wet or cold (or if you simply feel inclined to involve the 'bike in some way... the vibration of old British parallel twins has its points as far as the ladies are concerned), do make sure that the stand's up to the stress of two people plus some activity.

A broken motorcycle stand may not be top of the list for causes of coitus interruptus, but it's as effective as any of them, believe me!

Incidentally, if the car is the horseless carriage, is the motorcycle the horseless horse?

Back seat 69

Possible in most back seats (or of course on a front bench seat), though in narrower cars you'll need to keep the knees well tucked up. Either partner can be on top.
Just about impossible in an MGA. Back seat of Jaguar Mk 10 must be one of the best . . .

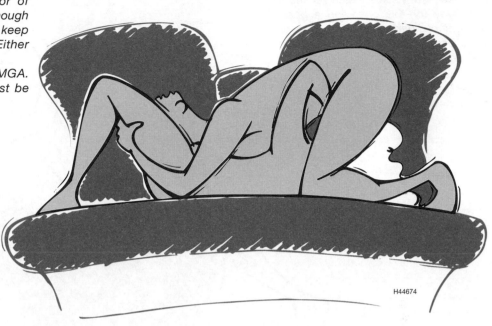

H44674

Sloping bonnet shuffle

Not recommended for owners of Mercedes, Jaguars or anything else with a protruding bonnet ornament (ouch). 2CV owners proceed with caution, the bonnet's not that strong. Ideally suited to Porsches, MGBs and the like. The woman can rest her feet on the bumper, or wrap her legs around the man's back as in the Climbing Vine position.

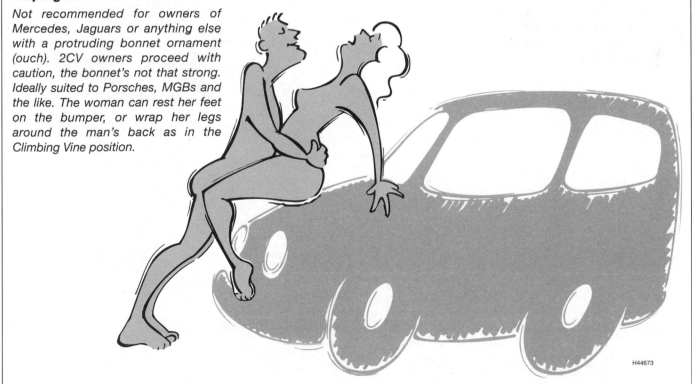

H44673

2

Morris missionary

You need front seats which recline a long way for this one, and a good amount of headroom helps. One or other partner may prefer to place their feet on the floor or on the dashboard.

H44671

Secret suction

One partner can perform oral sex on the other and keep below the line of sight; possible in virtually any car apart from a Messerschmitt.

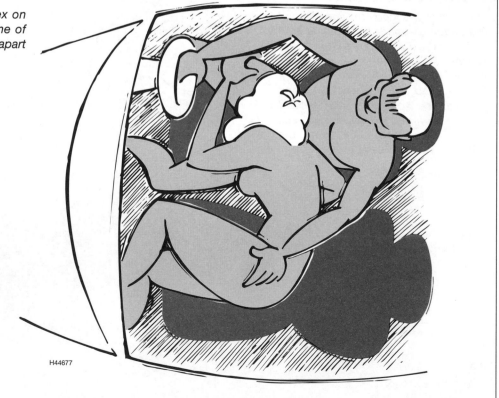

H44677

Sunroof special

The man kneels on the front seats, facing rearwards. The woman sits on the back seat and leans forwards to perform oral sex on him. (The sunroof may not be essential – it depends on the headroom, if you'll pardon the pun.)

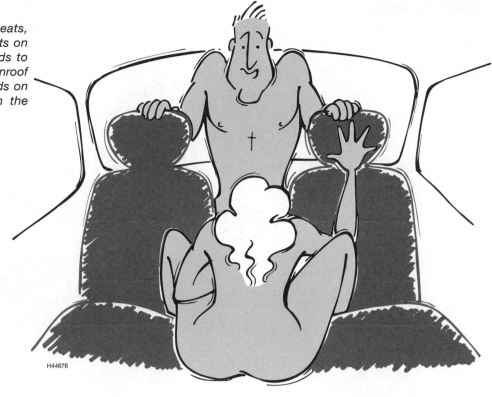

Ambassador

A variation on the Emperor position. The woman can press with her feet on the roof of the car to get more purchase.

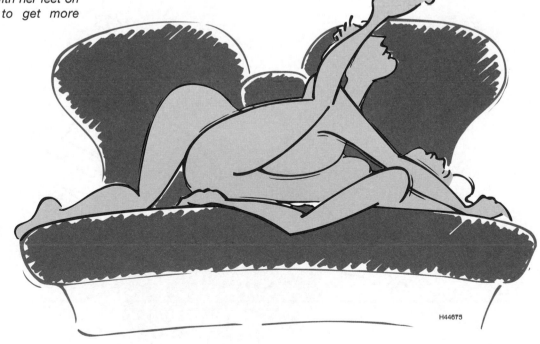

2

Horseless carriage

This is the Horse Riding position. Only works comfortably on the back seat in wide cars with lots of headroom, or in estates or vans with a mattress in the back . . .

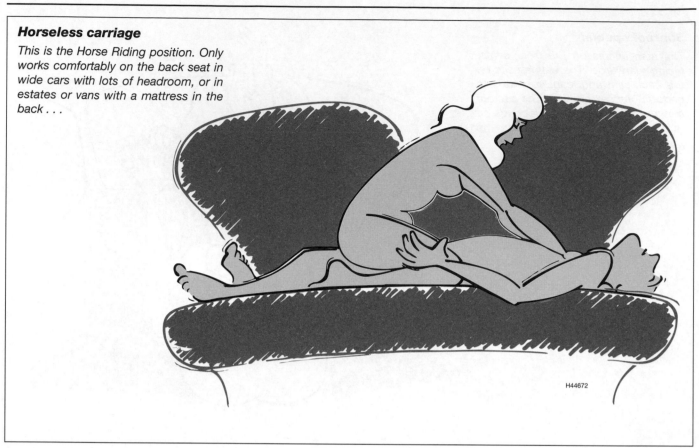

H44672

. . . but can also be performed in the front seat.

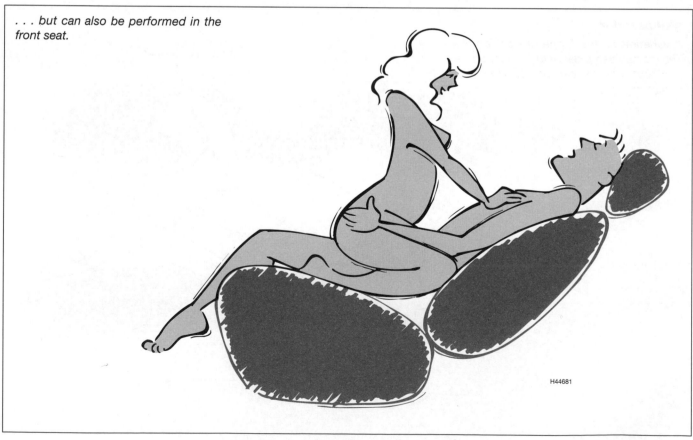

H44681

Wheelbarrow

No, it's not an old Skoda joke. The woman lies face down on the boot or the bonnet; the man supports her by the legs and enters from behind. Can be somewhat tiring, depending on the amount of lift required.

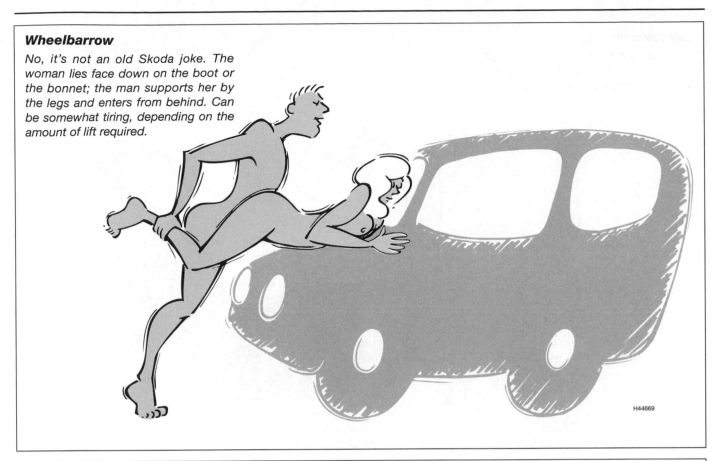

H44669

Nodding dogs

Doggie style on the boot or bonnet – but why stop there? Why not get up on the roof? Just be careful not to fall off.

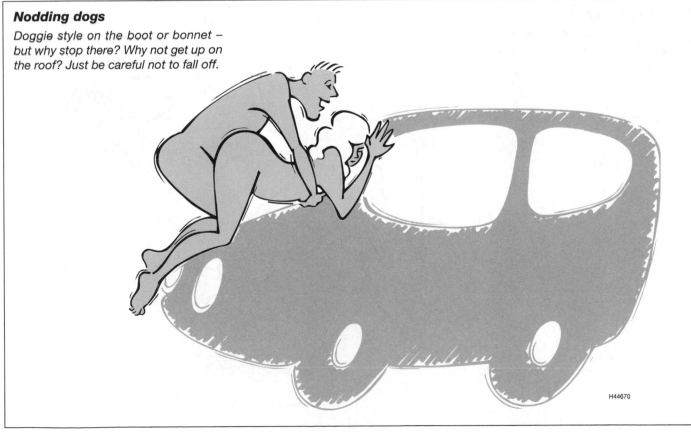

H44670

2

Lap dancing

Self-explanatory. You don't have to sit in the driving seat to do this – in fact it might be better if you didn't . . .

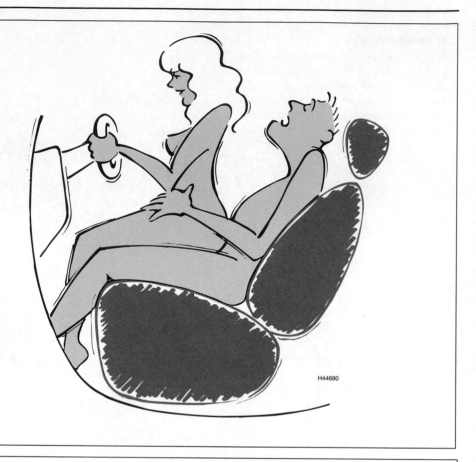

H44680

Woman on top

Another driving seat position. You'll be all right as long as the airbags don't deploy.

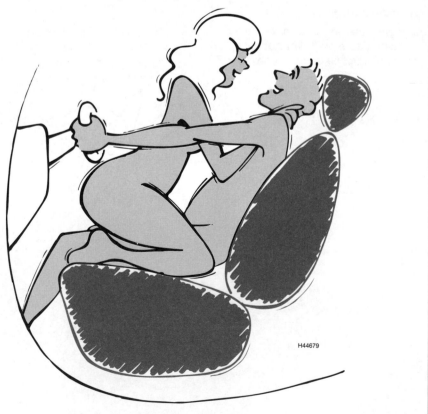

H44679

One in, one out

One partner sits sideways in the front passenger seat, with the door open. The other kneels or squats outside and performs oral sex on the one seated. The open door provides some protection from view.

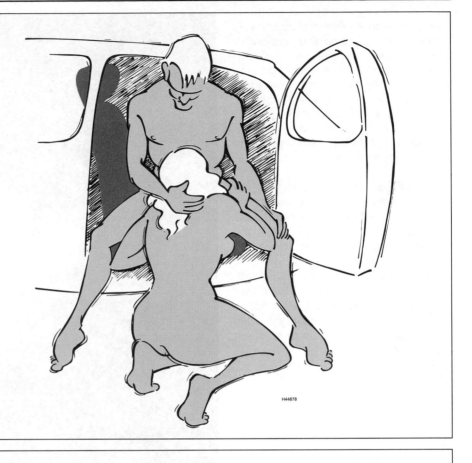

Hairpin bend

Another one for the bonnet or boot. The woman lies on her back and lifts up her legs; the man lifts her feet over his shoulders. Some height adjustments may be necessary – Citroën owners have the advantage.

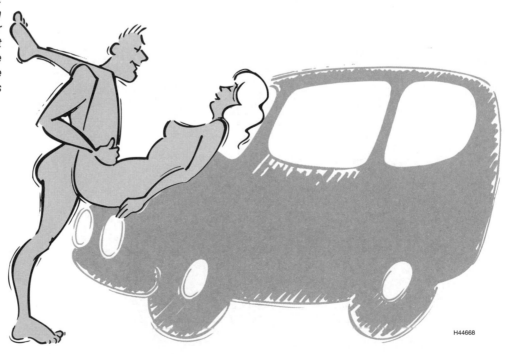

2

I recommend American or other luxury cars of the 50s and 60s, preferably with an auto transmission (column-mounted shift lever) and foot-operated parking brake, for maximum reproductive freedom in any position – bench seats, no seat belts or gear knobs to get in the way and no handbrake to need releasing in the heat of the moment.

The only drawbacks (apart from the running costs) are the over-large horn rings with which most of them are endowed, just ready to catch the unwary foot, bum, or whatever and attract the attention of the world to your activities. There is also the soft, super-bouncy suspension. Apart from the risk of sea-sickness, there's just no way you can pretend, if caught in the act, that you weren't up to anything untoward.

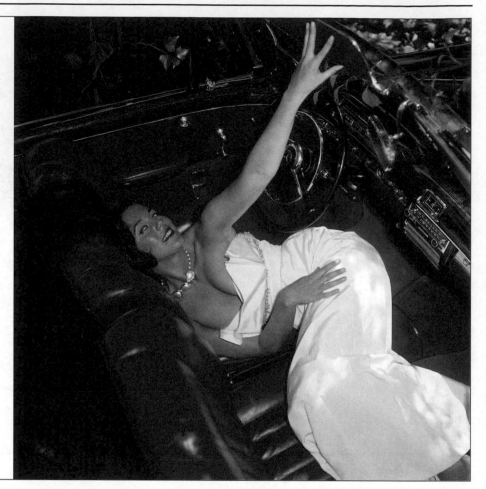

Chapter 3
Whatever turns your wheels

Contents

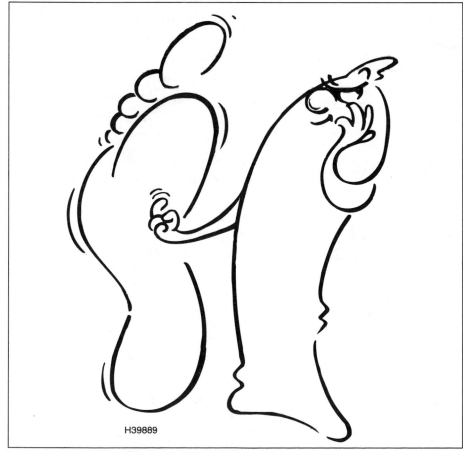

H39889

One person's fetish is another person's perversion

1 Fetishes

1 One person's fetish is another person's perversion. Have you ever wondered why there are so many fetishes? Why do people get so upset over things that turn other people on? It is pointless even trying to define a fetish because you will inevitably run into conflicts of interest. Perhaps we should stop trying to analyse what turns people on and simply lie back and enjoy it. Everyone has something which acts as a powerful sex stimulant, an object, smell or scenario. That's what makes the entertainment industry go round. It's a pity we can't be more honest with each other. Sex would be even more interesting.

Rubber duck

2 A fetish is only abnormal when it harms the person or those around them. Rubber fetishes are so

3

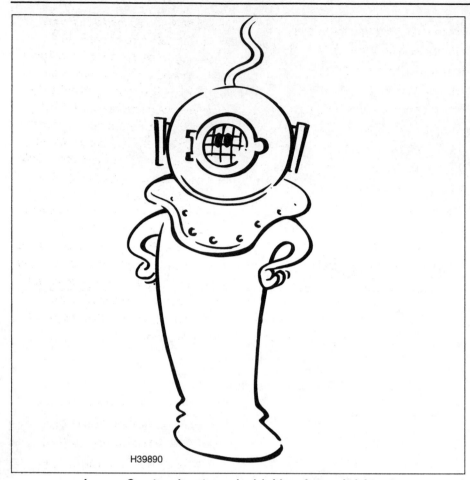

H39890

Jacques Cousteau is not everybody's idea of a good night out

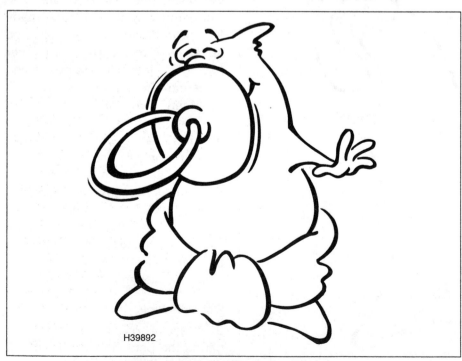

H39892

Being a baby is the ultimate in submission

common it can hardly be called abnormal but rather one end of a spectrum most people would consider unusual. This attraction towards rubber can be so strong it can almost supersede the attraction to people themselves. This limits the choice of sexual partners because making love looking like Jacques Cousteau is not everybody's idea of a good night out.

Dear Doctor

Please help. I have a problem which has been bugging me for ages. I love sex, but I really love sex dressed head to toe in rubber. It started when I was working in London and I met a girl who introduced me to the pleasures of rubber. I thought I'd found Heaven and we often indulge in sex in rubber which includes threesomes with women and men. I never thought of being gay, but when we're all dressed up I don't care who I'm making love with. Am I a freak to want to wear rubber suits and masks during sex?

When sex becomes so fixated and frenetic, safer sex can go to the wall and not for a knee-trembler either. Mixed couples for casual sex are potentially lethal without taking the correct precautions; consider covering yourself all over with rubber, and I do mean all over.

Happy nappy

3 Being a 'baby' is the ultimate in submission. You are totally dependent upon your 'mother' or

Dear Doctor

A few months ago I went around to my boyfriend's flat to give it a clean and tidy. While I was in his bedroom I discovered a hold-all containing large-size nappies, rubber pants, a feeding bottle and dummy. There were also some magazines with letters and photographs from people who dress up in this way. I was shocked to say the least. He'd never even hinted that he found such things a turn-on. I confronted him and eventually he admitted the truth, that he'd been dressing up as a baby since his late teens. We talked it through and came to a compromise, so now once a week I bathe him, put him in a nappy and rubber pants and bottle feed him. My problem is I've begun to enjoy mothering him and find myself looking forward to having him as my baby. Surely that can't be right? Do you think I should stop? I would appreciate any advice you can give me.

Along the spectrum of sexual pleasure you will find just about everything which turns people on. So long as it harms no-one and takes place between consenting adults there is no problem. Your boyfriend is enjoying one of the 'fringe benefits' of sex. If you enjoy the sexual play then fine. You may find it becoming tiresome and questions may come into your mind about the future should you wish to have children. If only for these reasons it would be best to continue to limit the amount of time spent in this form of sexual activity and to experiment with other, less personally-demanding activities. A great danger is to lose sight of the person you are so fond of in favour of your natural instincts as a potential mother. Be careful where you stick that nappy pin. You may both regret it.

'carer'. For some men this is linked to the only real happiness they can remember. As they grew up life became more challenging and harsh. They were not allowed to express their emotions by crying for instance. Dressing as a baby is predominately a male preserve, probably because of the way we bring men up to be dominant, expressionless, and never admitting they have a problem. Successful businessmen are among those who find this type of sexual behaviour a form of release from the straight-jacket of conformity imposed upon them by society.

Clothing maketh the man

4 Clothes are a powerful sexual stimulant. It is possible to 'fix' on some article of clothing which enhances sexual pressure. Shoes, underwear, hats, ties, belts, you name it and for some people they act like an aphrodisiac. If this fix becomes too powerful, it is impossible to have sex unless they are present. Some men for instance

Dear Doctor

My boyfriend and I have been together almost a year and love each other very much. We plan to get engaged at Christmas. I am rather worried as I think that I may have started him on a bondage fetish. To explain: we were larking about on the bed together and I was sitting on his back, the cord of his dressing gown was beside me and for a joke I pulled his arms behind him and tied his hands with it. He was struggling and yelling and I have to confess I was teasing him a lot. I even tied my tights over his mouth as a gag. I noticed that he had an enormous erection and, without going into the more sordid details, we had sex. Since that time, however, he has asked me to tie him up whenever we have sex and when I have refused he has got very upset. I am not a prude, but I would not be happy with our future love-making dependant on me trussing him up every time. I blame myself as, quite innocently, I did it for a joke, but it seems to have backfired on me. Is there anything I can do?

Sex can get pretty boring at the best of times. Doubly so if there is only one way to do it. Experimentation keeps sex lively but any form of sexual play, no matter how exotic runs the risk of familiarity. Where the fun is unequal, as in your case, one partner is bound, if you will forgive the expression, to get fed up. You need to shout, 'wot about the workers' very loudly in his ear, preferably while gagged. Using tights for partial strangulation is a dangerous manoeuvre, they can actually kill, do not use tights or nylons as gags either. They ladder easily unless your partner has taken his false teeth out first.

3

cannot sustain an erection unless their partner is wearing boots. This kind of fetish is not abnormal; it is simply one of the many things which makes sex more interesting. It was rumoured that one former government minister could only have sex while dressed in his local football team strip. For many people a clothes fetish enhances their pleasure from masturbation.

5 The hugely popular film, *A Fish Called Wanda* forever placed shoe fetish on the list of 'must do's'. Being a psychotic murderer is an optional extra. Shoes are a powerful attractant for some men, which explains why women hobble around on otherwise illogical stiletto heels. Feet are actually very sexy. Toe sucking is considered a major turn on, not least by some former members of the Royal Family. It's called 'shrimping' after the appearance of the little toe. Toe sucking probably has its roots in infancy when your parents pretended to bite your toes off or subject them to 'this little piggy'. Shoes simply enhance the allure.

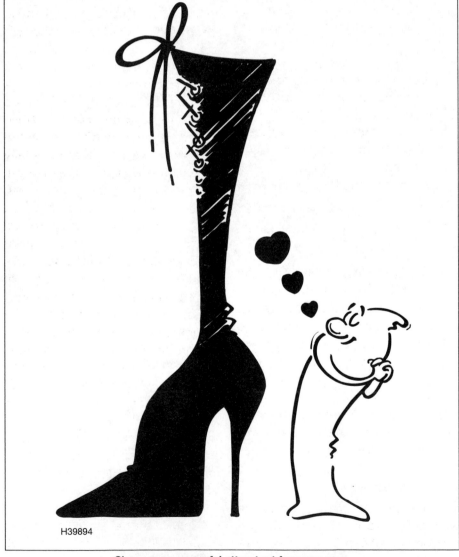

H39894

Shoes are a powerful attractant for some men

Dear Doctor

I have been with my boyfriend for some months and we seem to hit it off very well and when we have sex he is very gentle and considerate. But I have recently discovered he has a shoe fetish. We had been out to a disco and on our return I went to make some coffee leaving him watching the TV. As the door was ajar, I glanced into the living room and was stunned to see him with one of my boots over his nose. I could not fail to see that he had a huge erection which he was masturbating furiously. I tackled him immediately and to say he was embarrassed is putting it mildly. I managed to drag it out of him that he had a thing about my footwear and especially my boots. As I really like him I agreed that I would wear my boots when we have sex although I feel foolish wearing my boots and very little else. On the plus side I have to admit that our sex has improved a lot. I have been considering asking him to consult a sex therapist but quite honestly I don't know how he would take my suggestion. I would not like to give him up as I have very strong feelings for him.

Being the sole of discretion I can tell you that this is quite common amongst men. We also know that pheromones, the sex attractants, are probably secreted through the feet as well as elsewhere.

2 Groups

Pick a number, any number

1 Is it possible to be faithful yet unfaithful? For centuries men have rationalised that it is quite

Dear Doctor

I accidentally came across a book in my husband's possession which featured letters from husbands who got turned on by watching their wives performing with other men. I was shocked, and when I confronted him he admitted that he'd often fantasised about this. We are both dark-haired and my husband said he would really get turned on at the sight of me giving oral sex to a very blond man. I am totally confused! Does my husband really love me? Could he be bisexual? Should I please him by fulfilling his fantasy? I could just about do so, I think, provided the person was a total stranger, clean and very attractive! Help!

No, he is neither gay nor abnormal. Such fantasies are popular as shown by the magazine you accidentally found belonging to your husband. Even so, fantasy turned into reality can be a great disappointment. You may find it better to help him enjoy the fantasy rather than the reality. Talking through such an encounter can provide great sexual stimulation without the hassle of divorce. Either that or get him to buy a blonde wig.

reasonable to employ the services of a prostitute while away from their partners. Few women would subscribe to this philosophy. Yet there are couples who find the idea of group sex, 'controlled infidelity' very exciting.

Three's a crowd and four is even better

2 What generally happens is one partner enjoys it more than the other and wants to continue. Jealousy starts to creep in and then comes the full blown row. Do whatever you both want to do so long as nobody gets hurt. There are clubs which cater for couples, most people go along as spectators. If you can survive this experimentation you have an extremely stable relationship. Most marriages and relationships eventually crumble. Safer sex is vital. And don't forget where you leave your socks – verrucas are such a nuisance.

3 One of the truisms of any long standing relationship is you need to work at it. Familiarity begins to equate with boredom. Finding new and exciting things to keep the sparkle in your love life is one of the keys to a successful sexual relationship. In these days of sexual liberation it can sound prudish to advise caution. Even so, fantasy turned into reality can be a great disappointment. The single biggest danger is jealousy. Some couples appear to survive these experiments but for some it is the last straw and they drift apart.

Room with a view

4 Some couples video themselves in action. This is not new. Many a bedroom has been built with a mirror over the bed and many a book has

been written about them. We are fascinated by the sexual antics of ourselves and our partners. This can spill over to wanting the voyeur's view of the action. Unfortunately this can go horribly wrong when one or other of the couple like what they see too much.

3 Libido

1 There still exists great confusion over a lack of libido and impotence. Similarly, drugs like Cialis, Viagra or Levitra are often misconstrued as aphrodisiacs. Not so. You still need all the normal arousal before they will work. Loss of libido is the lack of sexual drive, while impotence is the inability to maintain an erection. A man can have a raging libido but be unable to have an erection. While impotence can very often be treated with drugs, loss of libido is usually more complex and drugs feature very rarely. Part of the problem with unfulfilling sex is expectation which is not helped by the media portrayal of sex as always involving an orgasm and a major contributor to noise pollution. Not achieving an orgasm and enjoying sex more in tune with 'Silent Night' rather than the Brandenburg Concerto can lead to feelings of inadequacy. Young men and women are often absolutely obsessed with being a 'normal sexual being' and seek reassurance through magazine and web site agony columns which unfortunately run 'wham, blam sex' articles at the same time as giving quite reasonable advice.

2 Most obstacles to enjoying sex are psychological and environmental. Being constantly tired is not a good

3

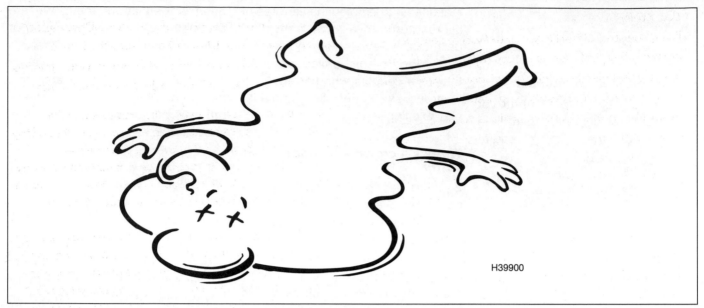

H39900

Impotence is the inability to maintain an erection

Dear Doctor

I often wonder if there is such a thing as female impotence? I am a woman aged 27 and I've been having difficulty coming to terms with my problem, which is lack of sexual appetite. This problem started long before I can remember. A couple of years back I informed my GP who recommended a psycho-sexualist, but after a couple of sessions and advice on masturbation I opted out as my situation didn't improve. I have had casual relationships but I simply cannot feel any emotion and therefore do not get aroused. I remember feeling the adrenaline flowing through me in my teen years. I remember in those days I was very sexually active and responsive. My current situation has made me promiscuous in the hope that I'd finally break through the 'barrier'. I wonder if it is a mental or a physical problem. Am I incapable of love, or impotent – if there is such a thing – or more likely sexually dead. Please help me.

  PS I can assure you I'm heterosexual and would never consider myself even a bisexual.

The good news is you once were easily sexually aroused, so all the equipment appears to be in working order. Most problems with sexual appetite are caused by tiredness, alcohol abuse, anxiety or poor stimulation. All of these can be helped once the problem has been identified.

  You may be confusing 'love' with sexual desire. Equally you may be trying too hard and are having sex with men you don't find in the least bit attractive. Sexual play from someone who really turns you on is worth two in the bush, as it were. Keep the dangers of casual sex at the front of your mind and always insist they wear a condom. There are female versions available.

recipe for sex. Similarly, having kids asking for drinks of water during the juicy bits doesn't help much either.

3 Deficiency of hormones such as thyroxin, which governs the body's metabolic rate, can drastically reduce libido. Your GP can check these out but you should eliminate the obvious factors first.

4 Thankfully there is still mystery in sex and human attraction. We are attracted to different people for different reasons. Despite all the attempts by the media to tell us what is and is not sexually attractive in people, we still have an enormous range of preferences. Which is good news for the diversity of the human species.

5 Libido is not constant throughout life. Nor is it the same in every person. Work often gets in the way of sex. Worries over promotion, redundancy or friction between people you work with can all directly affect your sex drive. At the end of the list come physical problems.

Dear Doctor

I'm 40 years old and have only had two sexual partners. The first was six years ago at which time I lost my virginity. I waited for 34 years only to be very disappointed. This relationship lasted only a few days. My only first, real boyfriend was four years ago and I went out with him for two months. We had sex within the first week. I was so naive because my partner would not wear a condom. I allowed him to have unprotected sex. I thought it was love and became really hooked on this man but I later learnt that he only went with me because of my large chest. I think I maybe only went out with him because I was pleased that he had asked me out. I worry that I may never have a real, normal relationship. I'm not really bothered about sex – I don't really enjoy penetration but I would like companionship – love without sex – am I normal? I would also like to add that I feel socially awkward and find it difficult to make friends with either men or women, in fact I am quite a loner.

You are perfectly normal. One of the problems with our hyped society is everyone is expected to not only desperately want sex every minute of the day but also to be able to provide it as often too. In truth people's sexual appetites vary considerably. People are attracted to other people for lots of reasons and it would be difficult to say what is 'right' or 'wrong'.

You are quite correct to be concerned over unprotected sex with people you know little about. Vaginal sex is not so hazardous as anal sex but still carries a significant risk. Non-penetrative sex can be every bit as exciting and is far less risky. If your boyfriend wants penetrative sex and so do you, make sure he uses a condom. Either that or a cold shower.

6 Boy George once said he would rather have a cup of tea than sex. In fairness, there are those who would rather have a cup of tea than Boy George…

normal body function should ever have raised such alarm. Things are changing but there still lingers a taboo over body functions which are pleasurable. Things were worse, much worse, in the recent past. Victorian boys caught masturbating had long safety pins pushed through their foreskins. Not only did this make erections extremely painful, it

4 Masturbation

1 Men are generally less able to discuss psycho-sexual matters and commonly use different expressions to describe sex organs, masturbation and intercourse itself. Not surprisingly, the list of euphemisms for male masturbation is almost endless. Five knuckle shuffle, Ham Shank, J. Arthur Rank, Hand Shandy, Barclays' Bank etc. Women do not have the same range of vocabulary in this area. This probably also reflects the fact that it is only relatively recently that female masturbation has been recognised and accepted.

Masturbation mantra

2 Masturbation is normal. It is difficult to explain why a perfectly

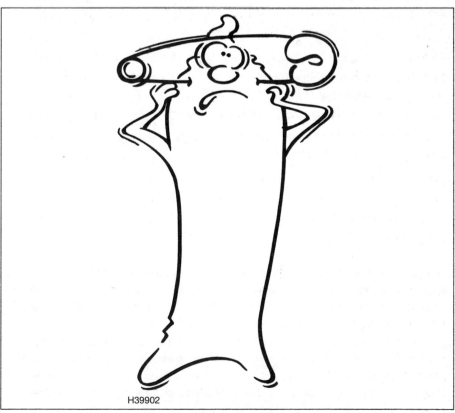

H39902

Victorian boys had long safety pins pushed through their foreskins

3

made even thinking about masturbation a bad idea. Why society should be so much against what is essentially a harmless, even beneficial exercise, is difficult to fathom. Population control is a recent phenomenon. Most societies used to actively encourage large families with tax incentives or prizes. Wasting sperm, and perhaps more to the point, the sexual act itself, was seen as more than just being antisocial. The Talmud clearly states, 'Thou shalt not practice masturbation either with hand or foot'. This may simply be a way of preventing dislocated hips. The Bible comes down pretty hard on masturbation. Corinthians just hates waste. 'Be not deceived. Neither fornicators, nor effeminates, nor abusers of themselves... shall inherit the Kingdom of God'. Must be quite lonely up there.

3 Doctors must be chaste, generally these days by solicitors. Insanity was closely linked to masturbation. Even worse, it heralded the end of civilisation as we knew it. In 1850 the New Orleans Medical and Surgical Times reckoned it was a danger to be rooted out. 'Neither plague, nor war nor smallpox, nor a crowd of similar evils have resulted more disastrously for humanity than the habit of masturbation. It is destroying the element of civilised society.' In those days the very last person you talked to about masturbation was your doctor, especially if he happened to be holding a large pin.

Masturbation myths

Sperm builds up in the testicles so it must be released on a regular basis

4 Sperm are produced by the testes and are carried by the vas deferens to the prostate at the base of the penis. The bulk of material actually ejected comes from the prostate, epididymal and Cowper's glands, not from the testis. Sperm are produced at a more or less constant rate and stored for a short while in the epididymis. Any that are not ejected are reabsorbed and recycled. Similarly for the rest of the secretions.

Masturbation can affect your eyes/ears/skin/brain

5 Fortunately untrue otherwise the NHS would be in even greater trouble from overload. Deafness and

Dear Doctor

We had a discussion at our college about sexuality and were surprised to find a high incidence of masturbation among the girls here. The boys are surprised because they thought girls did not do this because they have no reason to masturbate. 'Boys have to masturbate regularly because of the build up of seminal fluid. Girls do not have this problem.'

Two questions:
- Is female masturbation common?
- Why do we girls needs to masturbate?

If ever there was a golden excuse for having a five knuckle shuffle, the dreaded 'build up of seminal fluid' has to be the best yet. The testicles of boys not masturbating on a regular basis will not explode, showering your classmates with genetic material. The reason why both men and women masturbate is simple: it's great fun.

poor vision are not recognised complications of masturbation. On the other hand, painful ears when your dad finds you with his 'adult' magazines most definitely is.

All in the mind

6 Most men use visual stimulation while most women use fantasies instead. These can involve all kinds of weird and wonderful combinations that most people would never normally admit to. Sex with multiple partners, well known figures, partners of the same sex and especially film or television personalities. This may not extend to politicians.

7 Around 15 to 20% of women routinely use 'sex toys' such as vibrators which are available from most sex shops. For obvious reasons they are invariably battery driven. Shapes vary. Designs loosely fashioned on the penis are still popular but torpedo-shaped vibrators with warty protuberances are gaining ground. Even round ball-shaped machines can be purchased. Although the risk is less than penetrative sex, it is possible to transmit sexually transmitted diseases through a shared vibrator. Either cover it with a condom or wash it thoroughly between each person. It might be a good idea to switch it off before trying to slip the condom on. Such is their acceptability in polite society, the Family Planning Association (FPA) runs a mail order service.

8 One great innovation is the increasing use of mobile phones switched to vibrate mode. Your lover can ring you to tell you how much they love you, literally. Unfortunately no telephone company, including by way of irony Nokia, has investigated the effect of high frequency radio waves on the vagina. Until this evidence is available caution must be advised, not to mention washing your hands after making a call.

5   S & M (sadomasochism)

1   Sadomasochism evokes powerful indignation. Rightly so when it involves people who do not want anything to do with it. It can be argued, and it often is, that sex itself is a form of sadism and masochism. All kinds of games that nobody likes to admit to can take place behind those net curtains. The spectrum is considerable, from verbal pain to physical. Being 'hurt' in a controlled fashion with the ability to see the need to stop the process is fundamental to human behaviour. 'Adventure' is often just another word for near self inflicted torture. Who in their correct tiny minds wants to be spunaround, shaken up and down and subjected to horrific visual displays? Nip down to your local funfair and see them queuing up for 'joy rides' which are guaranteed to shake your ear lobes off. Or anything else which is hanging down for that matter. Maintaining that fine line between what is acceptable and ethically correct and personal gratification can be easy to step over. Freedom comes at a price.

Balancing act

2   The big danger is going too far or getting carried away. Make sure that you have a code word which you both recognise as being the end of the session. Choose one that is

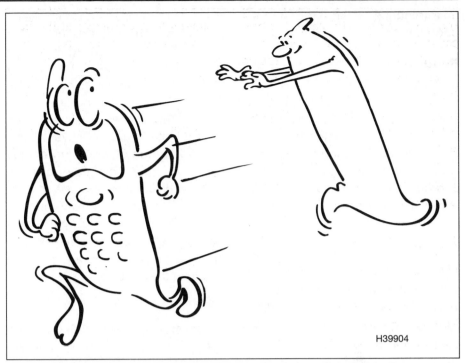
H39904

One innovation is the increasing use of mobile phones switched to vibrate

Dear Doctor

I am a 40 year old man and admit to liking having my bottom spanked. I understand that this is not uncommon amongst men. Not long ago I met a woman about my age and admitted my fetish to her. She then told me how she had been slippered at school on her bottom and despite the pain, it had not been an altogether unpleasant experience. What concerns me is that she wants me to take this further and hurt her quite severely. For instance, a few days ago she produced a cane and asked me to give her a number of hard strokes with it. The thing is, I was caned across my bare bottom at school and it's not something I would want to subject a woman to. Is this something I should put a stop to, or is it harmless? Also, is it common for women to like this sort of thing?

You have obviously met someone who is fairly close to your way of thinking when it comes to enjoying sex. She, however, wants to go a bit further than you are prepared to go. This is very common when it comes to matching each other's sexual expectation. So long as neither of you is mentally or physically injured and that you both recognise the danger of physical excess then there should be no problem. Make sure that you have a code word which you both recognise as being the end of the session. It is difficult to give you strong advice and it really does depend upon what you both feel about your expectations. You need to talk to her and explain your worries. Point out that you are unhappy when it comes to actually hurting her and that you find it difficult to fulfil her wishes.

3

unambiguous. 'Stop, stop' is not a good choice.

Bondage

3 This type of fetish is very common with a broad spectrum, some of it taking place in public. The far end of the scale, with total immobilisation through bandages or rubber, represents the ultimate in submission and most people will experience minor variations on this theme, particularly as children. Being tied up is a childhood delight which also has its place in adult sexual play. Many transvestites prefer clothes which are ridiculously tight. They will tolerate bodices and corsets few women would entertain for a minute. It may all have a basis in the tradition of wrapping babies up very tightly. This may not have been very comfortable but it went with a lot of cuddles from mum or dad. There is a theory that mummification bondage may decline as parents are encouraged not to overheat their babies.

4 Never, ever put anything around the neck which could tighten. Similarly, gags should be loose, not prevent mouth breathing and not be inside the mouth. On a very serious note, never bind your chest, throat or mouth too tightly. Over-tight bandages will cause swelling which then tightens them even more. People, often young men, die from this form of sexual stimulation.

Painful relatives

5 Pain is relative and is actually part of sexual play. Having your back scratched with sharp finger nails may go down well during a steamy night's fun. You are not quite so sure when you have a bath or shower and you think someone has flayed your back with a cat o'nine tails. During many enjoyable or intensive acts, pain can be either disregarded or transformed into pleasure. How this happens is not exactly certain, and a lot of S & M addicts would pay good money to find out, but endorphins may play a role. These hormones are released from the brain and are involved in the perception of pleasure.

Dear Doctor

I have a rather peculiar and obsessive fetish which I think might be the reason for me not getting a girlfriend. This fetish is a strong form of bondage called mummification and not a single day goes past without a fantasy about being stripped naked by strict naughty nurses and then wrapped up in an infinite amount of bandages until my entire body is tight, white and completely immobile. How weird is this fantasy, and what does it say about my sexuality?

Resisting the temptation to discuss an Oedipus complex, this type of fetish is actually common. Your difficulty finding a girlfriend is perhaps understandable. I would suggest reading the contact pages of erotic magazines for a like-minded partner. You would need to take turns, otherwise your bedroom would very quickly resemble the British Museum Egyptology department. With about as much sex too. Unless you have a particularly understanding GP, it is unlikely you will get your bandages on the NHS.

Dear Doctor

I wonder if you can help me. The other night, after having sex, my wife and I started to discuss our fantasies. We shared lots of the same desires and want to try them, but my wife then said she wanted to be handcuffed to the bed while we made love. Is this normal? Should I go along with it – personally I'm not too sure.

Bondage is great fun so long as it doesn't get out of hand. Only use ropes which can be broken, handcuffs which have an emergency breakage built in and never, ever, tie anything around the neck. Not even in fun. We humans suffer badly from having our brains on the end of our necks and all the blood supply has to go through it to keep us from going cold. Strangulation is unfortunately not rare during sexual play. Agree on a code word which will instantly stop all bondage. There must be no confusion over the meaning of the word. 'Stop' is not the best choice as it tends to be muttered during the fun bits.

Crossing the line

6 Bondage is great fun so long as it doesn't get out of hand. Fantasy about rape is common but has no connection with the real thing. Men and women brutalised by rape suffer scars long after their tormentors have served their time. Between consenting adults, tying each other up allows an element of release from responsibility for their actions.

7 A fine line exists between enjoyment and fear. Even close, loving relationships can be brought into question when this line is crossed. If you find this hard to accept, try looking very closely at yourself in the mirror and make threatening faces. Unless you have a different type of mirror from mine, it can scare the pants off you.

8 Sometimes it is difficult to work out what is going on in a relationship. There can be a mixture of frustrated desires, mixed emotions and self doubt. Relationships, particularly sexual relationships, are never straightforward. Often one person wants to dominate while the other is submissive. Problems occur when both people want to take the lead role or both be submissive. Forget about men always being the master. Many happy relationships occur where this traditional view of sex is reversed. Similarly with gay men and lesbian

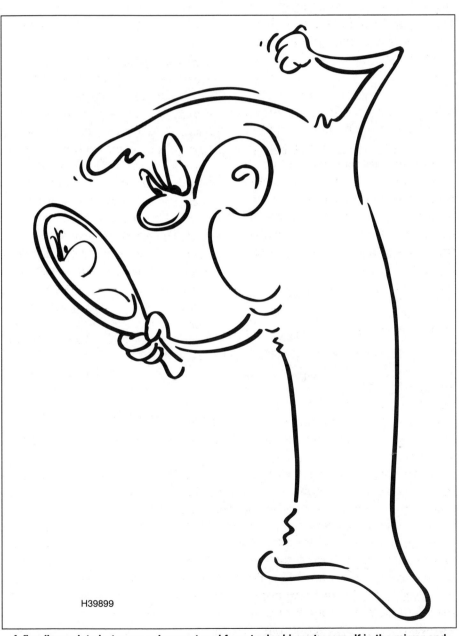

H39899

A fine line exists between enjoyment and fear; try looking at yourself in the mirror and make threatening faces

Dear Doctor

I am having serious sexual incompatibility problems with my wife. We've been married 11 years and I absolutely adore sex, whilst her sex drive is comparatively low. Consequently I have to make do with making love only when she wants – maybe 2 or 3 times a month. Added to this, I have an obsession with bondage and S & M – my wish is to be on the receiving end as the submissive rather than dominant partner. However, my wife views this kind of behaviour as perverted and unnatural and refuses to co-operate. As much as I love my wife, I am considering divorce as the only step towards sexual satisfaction. Can you offer any help or advice?

If only we had some sort of viewer's guide before we get hooked up to one person. Part of the problem is our innate inability to communicate better over areas we think of as embarrassing. Sexual preferences also change with time. Talking things through will often allow some kind of compromise. Finding something that she enjoys as well can allow you both to enjoy sex without it becoming the only way. Her concern will be that you will eventually only want one form of sexual pleasure, sadism and masochism. By convincing her that this should only be part of a much wider spectrum of sexual activity you might be able to experience what you desire. Her upbringing may also shade her view of such activity and imposing your wishes will only produce an equal and opposite reaction. At the end of the day compromise is the only way.

3

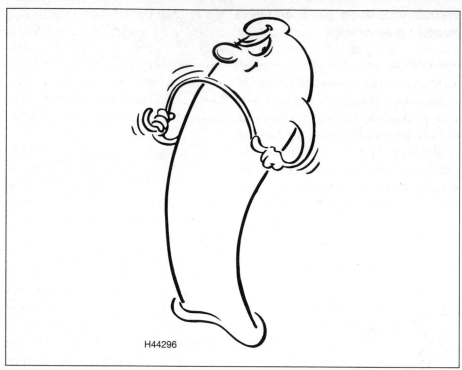

Teaching a younger person is a male and female fantasy

women. Teaching a younger person the art of sex is a fantasy of both men and women. Where would *The Graduate* be without Mrs Robinson? Northern Ireland's age for consent is seventeen as against Britain's sixteen. Can you be arrested on the boat from Liverpool just exactly midway in the Irish Sea? Most people lie in their bunks desperately wishing their partners could mind read. The rest are on the top deck vomiting into the prevailing wind.

6 Big boy's toys?

1 When it comes to sex toys, myths really take off. Like all contemporary generations young people like to

---

Dear Doctor

I have been with my boyfriend for almost a year and I love him very much and I know he loves me and our sex life is really great. However, something happened recently which really shocked me. I called at his flat unexpectedly after finishing work early and as I have

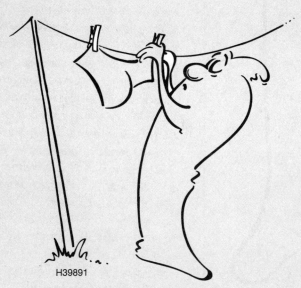

Make sure he washes your panties afterwards

my own key I let myself in. To my amazement I discovered my guy lying on the floor, his wrists and ankles were tied with my stockings and a pair of my panties were in his mouth. I thought for a moment he had been attacked and robbed. Then I saw he had a huge erection and had been masturbating himself. I untied him and he was very embarrassed and confessed that he had a fantasy that I tied him up and then used him as my sex slave. I never had an inkling that he was into this sort of thing and, quite frankly, I do not know exactly where our relationship is heading. I would welcome your advice.

This is the basis behind all answer phones, 'Sorry, I'm tied up at the moment. I'll get back to you'. This fantasy is common. He may well have wanted to be 'found out' so he could live his fantasy for real. He is basically offering you a chance to enter into this sex dreams. If you find the idea repulsive and cannot in any way take part, then say so. I suspect his ego and your relationship may well be a little crushed. Some fantasies can dominate all sexual play. If you are willing to take part, make it clear that you want your enjoyment too. Sex is a great bargaining tool. Make sure he washes your panties afterwards.

believe they invented everything, especially when it comes to sex. So some bad news for the latest generation – who will soon become the past generation – sex toys have been around for at least as long as bananas. Not that they have always been so publicly visible. Having sex toy shops on the high street, not to mention taking over where Tupperware parties left off, has raised their profile somewhat. Even so, we get so moralistic about such devices yet will happily use other machines to make our lives more pleasant in other ways.

Cock rings

2 Now here is a good example of an ancient sex toy. Cock rings are bands which fit around the base of the penis. They restrict the flow of blood back out of the penis thus making the erection firmer and more durable. Exotic variations on the theme include those with spikes, fur, or leather thongs which attach around the waist or neck. It can be tricky getting through the metal detectors at Heathrow airport while wearing one. Not a little embarrassing, too, although forcing a pilot to take you to Cuba on the basis of a threatening cock ring does stretch the imagination somewhat.

3 Only people with intact short-term memories should wear them, particularly if they are very tight (the rings, not the people). Leaving them on too long can cause the blood to clot inside the penis which doesn't give you a good erection so much as a very long black pudding. A particularly popular steel version, not for the faint hearted, has tiny needle points around the inside of the ring. Fitting these devices often prompts the exclamation, 'goodness me' or at least words to that effect.

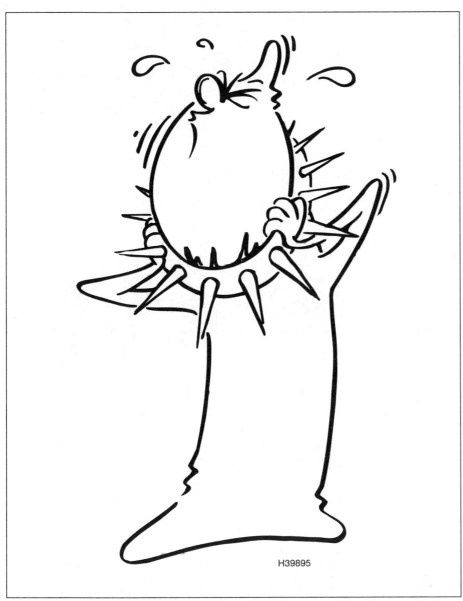

H39895

Exotic variations on the theme include cock rings with spikes

Dear Doctor
I don't know if this is a problem, but I like to use a cock ring while making love or even when I masturbate. I am 45 now and have been doing this for quite some time – I tried to stop but the feeling is so nice that I just can't. Is this normal and more importantly is it harmful? Can it damage my penis or my sperm? Should I make more effort to not use one, or try other toys?

No evidence is at hand to suggest that cock rings will put any strain on your sperm, excluding the need to jump through hoops, provided you don't keep them on too long. If you enjoy wearing them, and your partner has no objections, then there is little to lose from continuing to benefit from their use.

3

Things that go bump in the night

4 Nature seems to let us down at times. Things are not there when you need them and when they are they aren't big enough. Dildos are mentioned in ancient texts and archaeological digs turn up objects which were around way before people were planting potatoes. Tired men may have had recourse, not to mention frustrated women. Gay and lesbian magazines feature tried and tested shopping guides.

5 Size, as they say, is everything. Like teenagers with their first drink, there is a tendency to go for the Stallion Eye Water varieties in preference to more gentle, subtle and less thought-provoking machines. Go for the reasonable size first and work up. Fantasies involving female dominance over their male partner can come to grief with such overestimation of anal ring flexibility.

Pen is mightier than the toy

6 Not all toys are mechanical. In a sense literature and videos are a form of sex toy. There is a fine line between acceptable erotica and harmful perversion which damages either the subject or the user, or both. Nowhere can this be seen better than in paedophilia. Sadly, mainstream TV is not immune from accusing fingers. Portraying children in adult roles such as provocative 'pop idols' is dangerous stuff. We wrestle constantly with this in society.

7 Men seem to have a different view of erotic literature. Most men would not see a copy of Playboy as a co-respondent in a divorce trial. Women find them more degrading and threatening. When men are asked

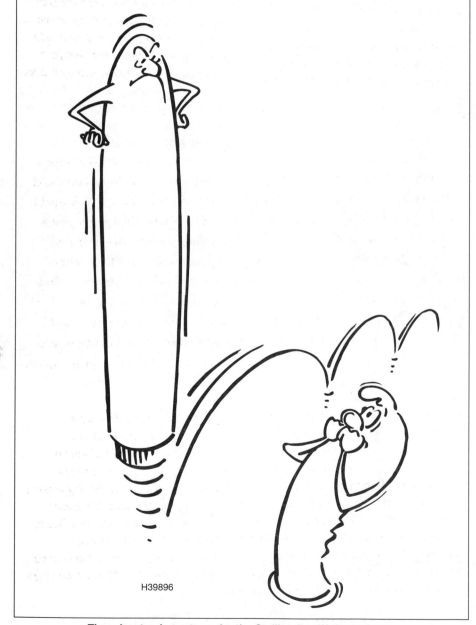

H39896

There is a tendency to go for the Stallion Eye Water varieties

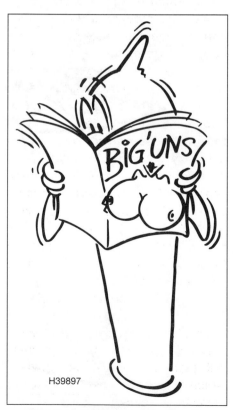

H39897

Men have a different view of erotic literature

Dear Doctor

After reading an erotic story in a magazine which she said turned her on, my girlfriend has expressed the desire to penetrate me using a strap-on dildo. She is often willing to help me with my fantasies so I am willing to give it a try. However, I am worried about the possibility of damage to my anus – the strap-on dildos that I have seen look enormous, and appear to be designed exclusively for female-to-female use. I have suggested that she could use a small dildo by hand, but she says that this wouldn't be the same at all, as the fantasy that she has in mind would not work for her that way. Please can you advise me about this. Are there any such devices on the market that are safer than others, and would my anus be permanently stretched by this type of penetration?

It won't be your anus that will be stretched so much as your sense of humour. When the anal ring was designed, poo of enormous dimensions had to be catered for. I am constantly amazed at the size of motions three year old children can produce when they really try. Unfortunately they also suffer occasionally from tiny anal tears which are painful when the next motion comes along. Repeatedly using a very large dildo could also damage the muscles surrounding the anal ring. Even so, gay men use this form of sex and there are few complaints of lax anal rings.

Interestingly, we use large dilators to treat recurrent anal fissures. Mind you, most people ask for a general anaesthetic before the operation is carried out. Perhaps you might happen to know a friendly anaesthetist who has been struck off recently. My advice is to use plenty of lubrication and take your contact lenses out in case your eyes pop.

about the same type of magazines for women they suddenly adopt all the attitudes displayed by women.

8 Part of the reason that sex toys are so emotive is the popular image of them as 'dirty' or 'kinky', yet they can also be seen as simply aiding people to do things in their sex life that they can either no longer easily do for themselves or can enhance what they are capable of doing. Those who are having trouble with their sight use 'seeing aids', usually called spectacles. If someone is having trouble hearing then a hearing-aid may be used, or artificial teeth by those who need help with eating and talking. It would therefore seem quite a natural progression to the idea of using a sex-aid for those who need some help.

9 Many of the items advertised in sex-aid catalogues are primarily for the purposes of titillation and some may find the catalogues offensive, but there are five or six devices which do have a prosthetic or therapeutic value.

Dear Doctor

I have been married for six years to a wonderful man. Last year I accidentally found some very explicit photos and videos that he'd obviously sent for and kept hidden from me. We discussed it and I said I didn't understand his need to look at these things. I agreed that he could have them, but I didn't want to know about them. Now recently, I've found more explicit photos along with a letter from a woman he's obviously been corresponding with for a long time. He is sending her money and she is posing for him and sending the photos. It hurts more now because it's personal and I feel like he's having an affair. Am responsible for driving him into this? I don't want to share him with anyone and I'm not giving up on the marriage.

It is not too late to sort things out. It is unlikely that your husband sees his relationship with someone supplying photographs as being unfaithful. He essentially is looking for excitement in his sexual relationship about which he fantasises regularly. Your confrontation convinced him that you would not be prepared to take part in his fantasies. Give and take is the order of the day when it comes to marriage or any form of relationship. Perhaps you should talk about your fears and inhibitions and let him explain his needs. Somewhere there has to be compromise, particularly if you are determined not to let your marriage crumble. On the plus side you could get him to pay you to pose for photographs for his personal use. Few charities would refuse this money should you wish to go non-profit making. This is a serious suggestion.

3

Chapter 4
Preferences

Contents

1 Sexuality

1 Women appear to come to terms with their sexuality far better than do men. More to the point they are able to talk to other women far easier than men can talk about being gay to other men. Some men agonise for ages before opening the closet door. Few are sorry they ever did.

2 Sexuality is a broad spectrum and it is possible, indeed common, for heterosexual men and women to be attracted to members of their own sex. This increases in certain situations where only the one sex is present. This does not make it right or wrong, it is simply an expression of human sexuality. In the rest of the animal kingdom such behaviour is also common. Whales in particular are known to have sexual play with members of their own sex. As the penis of the blue whale is at least six feet long this may explain that great spout of water which comes out of their heads. There is nothing to be ashamed of in investigating and examining your own sexuality. But be careful. Use safer sex and get in touch with a lesbian or gay helpline for some good advice. No matter how attractive you find Willie the killer-whale do not attempt under any circumstances to approach him without a 6 ft condom.

3 Thanks to all the pressures from society, parents and the law, people will try to rationalise their sexuality in bizarre ways. Instead of simply saying to themselves, 'I just so happen to like people of the same sex and find them sexually attractive' they will make up 'reasonable explanations'. This is also true of parents and society who will jump to conclusions such as upbringing or dressing the person as a baby in the wrong colour. Men try these mental contortions more than women, but both sexes produce some pretty weird interpretations of reality.

4 So otherwise where is the problem? The problem is with other people, girlfriends, parents, etc. Many men and women who eventually come out are pleasantly surprised at the reaction of their girlfriend/boyfriend when they tell them. They probably suspect anyway and may be attracted for exactly this reason. Parents generally go through a fairly

Dear Doctor

I have been thinking about having sex with another man for a couple of years now and I wonder whether I should go through with it. I love sex with women but a guy at work is gay and for some reason I really fancy him. I think he knows it because he is always smiling at me and it turns me on. Should I go for it at least once and see if I like it and what precautions should I take before allowing penetrative sex?

It sounds as though you have already made up your mind and that it is a case of 'when' rather than 'if'. You have probably noticed your attraction towards men from a relatively early age. But be careful – use safer sex.

4

predictable grief reaction. Disbelief, anger, guilt (did they make you gay?) and then coming to terms with the reality. Many parents not only continue to love their gay or lesbian children, they become fiercely supportive. There are some very famous bisexual people around. In truth for every famous bisexual person there are countless thousands of perfectly ordinary bisexual men and women living everyday lives.

5   Many women, like some men, find that they can still love someone without 'normal' sexual play. This tends to become more like sisterly love rather than that of true lovers in the sexual sense. Unfortunately for some women they confuse this with what is expected from a relationship without realising just how much they are missing. Awareness can then come gradually and not like a blinding flash of light. Recognising habit for what it is can be important for future happiness and fulfilment.

6   Men are generally aware of their sexuality fairly shortly after puberty and certainly by around 16 years of age. Men will bow to pressure from family and friends and go through heterosexual relationships just to 'fit in'. They may even marry and have a family. For some women this can take longer and many find themselves married, with children sometimes, before they understand their true sexual persuasion. Man or woman, it can be devastating for a marriage and cause pain on all sides. Lesbianism is not abnormal, nor is being a gay man. They are both parts of the spectrum of human sexuality which simply make us richer in our human resource for love.

Dressed to impress

7   Many people find this particular aspect of sexual enjoyment and personal fulfilment very attractive. Yet society can still be very harsh on people who commit the terrible crime of simply wanting to be who they are. If you feel more comfortable when you are dressed in the opposite sex's clothes then it

Dear Doctor

I am 25 years old and I've been with my boyfriend for 3 years. We both love each other very much but we haven't had sex now for nearly 18 months and this is worrying me very much. When we did have regular sex it never really did anything for me physically. I used to do it more out of habit than anything else, but now I don't like it if my boyfriend touches me intimately. I really love him, so why do you think this is? We still cuddle and are emotionally close in all other ways. Sometimes I wonder what it would be like to make love to a woman and images of naked women do turn me on. Could I be a lesbian? Being with a man does appeal to me even though the sexual desire isn't there. Please help.

You are starting to question your own sexuality. It is quite normal and common to have long-standing friendships, love included, with someone to whom you are not physically attracted. If you and your boyfriend are both happy with the situation, there is no problem.

Dear Doctor

I'm really worried about my sexuality. Please help. I'm a 19 year old male and I'm in a steady relationship with a woman. She is good looking and the most wonderful person. We have excellent regular sex and get on very well. The thing is, I masturbate up to three times a day and always fantasise about sexy muscle-bound men and I often stimulate my anus with a vibrator whilst fantasising that it's a man. I also look in the mirror and masturbate and find my own body very sexy indeed! My sister is a lesbian and when she came out my parents went mad. I've had feelings of being bisexual for years but I can't open up because my girlfriend would be so hurt. I'd love to go with a man but don't know where to find gay or bisexual men. Please help me as I'm so confused.

I don't think you are really confused so much as scared to come to terms with your own sexuality. Your sister's experience with your parents doesn't help matter much either. It's fairly obvious that you are either bisexual or gay. So where is the problem? The problem is with other people, your girlfriend, your parents and possibly your employer. Well actually that's really their problem not yours because you are what you are.

gives a good insight into your personality and you should not suppress it unless it brings you into conflict with people who are less understanding than your friends. Being honest really is the best policy.

Further information

8 If you would like to know more, look in the Contacts section at the back of the book.

Dear Doctor

I am a 26 year old male virgin and since I've lost my girlfriend six years ago I have lost all my self-confidence and my urge for sex. Since then I have started cross-dressing and I find that this relaxes me. My friends knew I was doing this for a while and now help me with my make-up and clothes. When I am dressed I look very convincing and raunchy. My problem is that I have met this girl who's interested in me but I don't know what to do or say to her. Should I tell her that I cross-dress or should I wait? I want to be totally honest with her.

PS I'm also very shy. What should I do?

Your new girlfriend probably recognises the way you feel more comfortable. You are very fortunate in having the support of your friends. You should tell your girlfriend how you feel. You may well be pleasantly surprised by the reaction.

2 On the small side

1 There is absolutely nothing wrong with finding people of short stature attractive. Ask anyone of short stature. Turn it on its head and ask is it abnormal for a person of short stature to be attracted to average-sized people. We all have the 'ideal' size in our heads. Generally speaking this is not absolute and many of us end up with partners different from what we consider our perfect match. The problem comes when only one trait is acceptable and becomes an obsession. People of short stature have as much right to a loving relationship with other people of whatever height. There is no law which says you must stick to people of your own physical build. Thank goodness or it would be a dull world indeed.

3 Healthy and gay

1 Disease has little concern for a man's sexual orientation. Life can be difficult for young men who are homosexual or unsure about their sexuality. Many feel like square pegs in round holes, driven by society, school, relatives and even the law. Some can become desperately lonely and depressed. Indeed the suicide rate is higher among gay teenagers. For most men, the process of 'coming out' is a difficult decision. However, they are often pleasantly surprised by the reception they receive from friends and family.

2 If you are not on a GP's list, you should register with one. Ask your friends, it is usually very obvious which GPs make a special effort or

Dear Doctor

Over the past year or so I have found myself more and more attracted to short women. To be more precise, people who would normally be called midgets or dwarves. Maybe it's because I feel they need protecting but I can't help but fantasise about having sex with a midget. To make matters worse, about two weeks ago I began to masturbate while watching my little sister's copy of 'Snow White'. I watch quite a lot now and I believe my mother suspects something. Apart from this, I'm a normal 20 year old who has no real vices. I don't think that this is normal behaviour and I don't think I'm gay – even though the blokes in the cartoon excited me. I need some advice. Is there any way to stop this?

There is nothing wrong about finding short people attractive. It may well be that you like to feel protective and in charge. You do need to decide whether you like small adults or if there is an attraction to small people because you perceive them as immature and child-like; this could be dangerous. I feel you may be confused over your own sexuality, as you deny gay feelings yet are attracted to short stature men. I would suggest a trip to your GP who could refer you for some psycho-sexual counselling.

4

Dear Doctor

I am writing because I don't know what to do. When I was 8 years old I started to dress up in my mum's clothes and one day I got caught. My uncle was very nasty to me because neither he nor my mum understood. My mum didn't speak to me for ages and threatened to tell everyone else if I didn't stop. I am now 26 years old. I have told my best friend and she is very understanding but I am very upset because I keep doing this bad thing and I can't stop. My friend asked me a lot of things about why I dress up, and I said I like to do it, I wish I was born a girl instead of a boy. I am very confused. I have thought of killing myself and just wish I could stop. I just want to wear women's clothes – is this such a crime? Please help me I don't know what to do.

First of all relax. You are in good company as cross-dressing is extremely common and is actually favoured in some societies. Austere clothing for men is a relatively recent phenomenon and when given half a chance men will be as flamboyant as women. For some people dressing as the opposite sex provides relief and sexual enjoyment. The desire to cross-dress for a transvestite or transsexual is very strong and many men have suffered ignominy and humiliation from a society more tolerant of violence than such a harmless act as cross-dressing. Parents often over-react in a desperate attempt to 'normalise' their child. It rarely works, causing only frustration, bitterness and desperation. It is important for you to come to terms with yourself as you are. There is nothing immoral, illegal or socially dangerous in being a transvestite or transsexual.

the use of clothes, make-up, etc, can give confidence and give you an opportunity to see life from a different perspective.

10 Being the in the wrong body is not uncommon and truly transsexual people are in no possible doubt that their bodies are of the wrong sex. They have all the emotional reactions, preferences, tastes and desires of the opposite sex and wish for nothing more than to live and be treated as members of the opposite sex. Genetics may not always be the single greatest factor: some people were treated by their parents from birth as if they were of the opposite sex, often because the parents wanted a baby of the opposite sex. This early environmental conditioning may be more powerful than the genetic influences. Transsexual people are often disgusted with the bodies they have to live in and may hurt themselves or even take their own lives. Suicide is far higher amongst this group than most others in society.

11 When it is fully established, by much psychological testing, that a person is genuinely transsexual, is suffering from no psychiatric disorder, and cannot ever be happy with the present anatomical sex, reassignment surgery should be offered.

Man-to-woman

12 The most common change is from male to female. It involves removal of the structures within the penis, but not the skin, reimplantation of the urine tube (urethra) to a place just within the new vagina, removal of the testicles and most of the skin of the scrotum, and the fashioning of an artificial vagina from the inverted skin of the penis, and labia minora from the scrotal skin.

13 This is not enough to create the female body so female sex hormones are given. These cause changes in the skin and hair and a re-distribution of fat on the hips, buttocks and breasts. Breast implantation (augmentation mammoplasty) is also often done. Although surgery is getting better all the time, the 'female genitalia' may not be quite perfect. Artificial lubrication is likely to be needed in the vagina and, as there will be a marked tendency to shrinkage, the use of dildos to maintain the shape of the vagina is often recommended. There is no guarantee that orgasm will be any more possible than it was before surgery. Even so for many people this is what they have desired all their lives and they are prepared to put up with what they consider minor problems.

Woman-to-man

14 Female-to-male surgery involves mastectomy to remove the breasts, followed by removal of the uterus and ovaries. Construction of a penis may then be attempted by grafting abdominal skin over a catheter. Unlike male-to-female changes, it is difficult to change the external appearance of the body although with subtle use of clothing there is often a convincing transformation.

nearly boil, then liqu
destroys the sting bu
quickly to avoid a stiff

4 Aromatherapy a
'aphrodisiacs'. The b
which is closest to o
pheromones' so this e
aftershaves or liberally
oil. Unfortunately the
versions tend to sme
surprisingly, like swe
soap-neglected groins
the smell merchants,
the point that no
pheromone' has yet
and may well turn out
reminiscent of ear v
human predilection for
people's ear lobes.

5 Spanish Fly is w
reputation and acts b
mucous membrane linii
the penis. It is a highly
derived from crushe
beetles. The itch persis
often driving the user
can also cause kidne
have died from this stuf
Cantharides beetles a
point out to humans t
evidence that their crus
as an aphrodisiac. Fe
science, however, they
give it a try the other wa

6 Repeated sex par
have a similar effect th
irritation. With an ex
panky the urethra, the
through the penis, a
glands and muscles v
it, become slightly i
acts as a stimulant an
go again.

7 Oysters are said
female genitalia a
aphrodisiac propert

Chapter 5
Orgasms

Contents

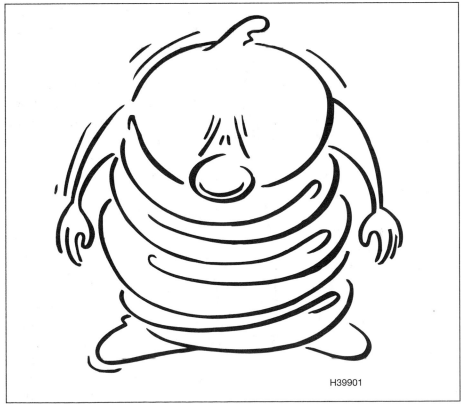

H39901

Sex with the long-awaited 'right' person can be bitterly disappointing

1 Did the Earth move?

1 Who ever coined the phrase 'and the Earth moved' has a lot to answer for. Losing your virginity is portrayed as a great mind boggling event which leaves you panting in orgasmic shock. Actually most people think, 'Is that it?' after their first penetrative sex. It is usually, by definition, a big anti-climax. Some people are lucky. For them the earth really did move, or had they simply forgotten to apply the handbrake on the Mini? It's not only the casual one off affair either. Some people, more often women, wait until they have met the 'right' person only to be bitterly disappointed with their first sex. Well the good news is, it gets better. But like playing the piano, practice helps.

5

2 One of the prob
hyped society is
expected to not on
want sex every minut
also to be able to pro
too. In truth people's
varies considerably.

Dear Doctor

Recently I've been h
sex with a very clos
mine. We aren't goin
couple even though
my hardest. My pro
that I have between
orgasms each time
love. I'm not joking.
tell me I'm the luck
in the world becaus
don't have nearly a
me. That's why I'm
it normal to have a
orgasms as I do, or
abnormal? Is it bec
friend of mine's per
inches long when f
and it gets right to t
He is the most gorg
have ever seen and
sight of him as wel
of him turns me on.
me. I am desperate
am normal.

Who cares. I'm already
with half the population
There is no such thing
number of orgasms du
intercourse. Personally
worry too much about
size or whether you are
would just lie back and
although it does explai
handwriting.

Dear Doctor

I am 25 and although while I'm having sex everything is fine, soon afterwards my penis becomes erect again without any stimulation and hurts intensely. So I have to have sex for a 2nd or 3rd time which is painful, until eventually I become flaccid. Because of the pain, I try to get it over with as soon as possible. Why is this? Would painkillers help?

Painkillers will do very little. What you are experiencing is probably the so-called aphrodisiac effect of urethral irritation. However, some sexually transmitted diseases, particularly non-specific urethritis (NSU), can have a similar effect. A visit to the local genito-urinary clinic (GU or GUM clinic) may be in order, especially if there is any discharge or rash.

ancient Romans transported enormous quantities from Colchester to Rome. The Emperor Vitellius ate up to 1000 at each sitting. Global warming is having an effect on our sex lives, if only in that Northern Ireland is now one of the major producers of exported oysters, modern Colchester being more than a tad further away from the sea than in Vitellius's time.

3 Female orgasm

1 Myths surround the female orgasm and it is heavily flavoured by romantic fiction. The most common myth is that the female orgasm is always both effortless and stunningly pleasurable. There are also minor

---

myths which are perpetuated in the media, such as:

- Climax follows climax.
- They are always easy to achieve and require no foreplay or romance.
- Penetrative sex is always necessary to achieve orgasm and the woman's climax should always happen simultaneously with that of her partner's.
- Female ejaculation – where something is released during the climax not unlike a fire-extinguisher going off – is commonly cited in erotic books but can be difficult to establish as fact.

2 The truth of the matter is quite different. Although the myths at first appear more attractive, by understanding the enjoyment of your partner and yourself, fact can be better than fiction.

Facts

- Most women do not always find it easy to achieve orgasm but it generally gets easier as they get older. Techniques and short cuts are learnt and used to greater effect.
- Foreplay is important. Yes, some people can climax very quickly but for most women it takes around 10 to 15 minutes.
- Physical stimulation is important. Few people can climax just by thinking about sex, which is great news for school teachers of adolescent boys.
- While it can be very pleasant for both parties to climax at the same time, most people do not.

3 The media would have us believe that you are a failure if you cannot have multiple orgasms. Worse still, you are a complete and utter failure if

---

you cannot have any kind of orgasm at all. Neither of these is true.

4 Familiarity doesn't breed

1 Men are often driven to distraction or to near exhaustion trying to bring about a climax for their partner. We tend to lay an enormous emphasis on the orgasm

Dear Doctor

I cannot achieve an orgasm with my present boyfriend, a condition which is a repeat of the situation which existed in my previous two long-term relationships, including my marriage. I have never experienced any sensation on vaginal intercourse but initially, at the beginning of these relationships achieve mini-orgasms from clitoral contact during heavy petting with my partners, but which always tends to decrease as the relationship with my partner continues. I love him so much but I feel too embarrassed to go to my doctor.

It is unlikely that there is anything medically wrong with you. Longer and more adventurous foreplay, along with experimentation, will help you keep your sex life exciting. There is no shortage of erotic literature which you can use with your partner to spice up your relationship. There are books full of good suggestions: The Big O by David Devlin and Christine Webber or Making the Honeymoon Last by Suzie Hayman, to name but two.

and fail to recognise that many women do not have an orgasm, or that their number and quality vary both between women and their partners. It is unlikely that there is anything medically wrong with a woman experiencing this. Familiarity, however, tends to bring in boredom and predictability with a declining sexual stimulation as you get to know your partner. This is part of the predictability which unfortunately tends to take over as time goes by.

5 Birthdays and orgasms

1 The average life expectancy for women is now around 80 years. It is perfectly reasonable to expect a good sex life well into old age, even if not quite the same as it was when younger. Boredom is a great killer of sexual play. Predictability, familiarity and lack of something new can lead to a stilted sex life. Some men, for instance, find naked women less sexually attractive than when they are dressed in evocative clothes. The fashion industry has not been slow to pick up on this. Obviously the same can apply the other way round. Many men hide their erectile dysfunction (impotence) by blaming it on their partner's decreasing attractiveness as they get older. Communication is vital.

2 Much as it hurts to admit it, orgasms for men can get more difficult to achieve as we get older. We do not really know why, and it is difficult to separate physiological reasons from psychological. Some men are simply quite happy with one orgasm per month when they reach the age of 70, but others expect the same kind of sexual pleasure they

Dear Doctor

I am writing to you in sheer desperation, hoping you can help. I am 61 years of age and my husband and I have been married for 41 years. Sex has never been very great and, although he is generous in many ways, he shows me very little love and affection. I did leave for 5 months a couple of years ago but we got together again. He can't seem to let himself go or talk to me when we're having sex (about 5 times this year so far) The other night when I got undressed I stood naked for a short time and he just lay there. I said, 'You don't take any notice of me nowadays, do you?' and he said, 'Well, you've got so fat'. I am 5'2" and 12 stone, and, yes I struggle but don't consider myself too bad. I cry myself to sleep and when I ask him to make love his answer is always 'I will if you want me to'. I feel I have been denied a full love life and feel very angry. I've even taken HRT to remain sexy and moist for him. Perhaps at my age I shouldn't have these needs. What can I do?

It is difficult to see both sides of the story when I only have your letter to explain what is happening. While I am not condoning your husband's behaviour there may be reasons and explanations other than he simply no longer cares about you. Perhaps you need to put some zing back into your relationship. Many men hide their impotence by blaming it on their partner. By saying you are too fat he may be scared to tell you that he can no longer sustain an erection. Communication is vital as these kinds of running sores can lead to a break up in the relationship. At the end of the day this may be all you can do if you wish to have a better life and you are still young enough to do it.

had in their teens. In truth most men develop better control over their orgasms which is much appreciated by their partners. (See *Impotence/ erectile dysfunction.*)

3 There are ways of improving your chances of having orgasms later in life. Simply being fit and not overweight are important. Not smoking and cutting back on saturated fats also makes good sense, as both are linked to erectile function. Keeping boredom out of the equation is the single most important factor. Once sex becomes predictable and too familiar it can be difficult to have so many orgasms as when you first met your partner.

4 Missing out on your sex life can be caused by a whole battery of things, not just age. Generally speaking if there was a problem at the onset it will take some work from both partners to improve matters. This is often easier said than done.

6 Types of orgasm

Female orgasms

1 A great deal of fuss is made about whether G spot orgasms are better than clitoral orgasms. Freud, the father of psychoanalysis, reckoned clitoral orgasms were for teenagers while the vaginal versions

5

were for mature women. We now consider it probable that women will be able to experience both at any stage of their sexual development. Named after its 'discoverer' Ernest Grafenberg, the G spot is found somewhere on the front wall of the vagina. It can be found by gently stroking the upper/front wall of the vagina with a well lubricated finger. There is nothing to see. Don't expect a big sign with an arrow: G SPOT HERE. Women experience orgasm differently at different times of the month. This is often mirrored in the type of sex they would rather have. For some women the days immediately before a period are the most exciting and they seek mad passionate sex. Others would rather have a cup of hot chocolate and wonder why their partners are reading the newspaper in the shower.

Male orgasms

2 Men are supposed to also have the equivalent of the female G spot. It is said to be found on the rectal side of the prostate. As bad luck would have it, the only way of getting at this particular part of the male anatomy is either with a finger in the anus or by major surgery. What we do know is that men can have an orgasm without any physical stimulation – wet dreams were not a figment of your imagination – ask your mum. Generally speaking, however, men find it much easier if there is mechanical stimulation of the penis or anus. This can be achieved with either sex toys, themselves or someone else.

3 If you are a woman, never trust a man if he tells you that he can climax without actually ejaculating. This is the equivalent of having a baby without ever being pregnant. And you will find out just how very true this is in about nine months time.

4 Even vibration from travelling in a car can produce an erection and possibly orgasm. Long distance lorry drivers call it Diesel Dong. As it happens Diesel, the designer of the engine after his own name, committed suicide by throwing himself off a ship. Perhaps he knew what else his name was going to be attached to. Cynical women would say this just goes to show how much men can fall in love with their cars. Simple friction against an inanimate object will suffice although the human variety works better. This is the basis behind frottage where men, and to a lesser extent women, derive sexual pleasure from rubbing themselves against people in tubes and buses.

5 Working out face down on a bench can produce the same effect,

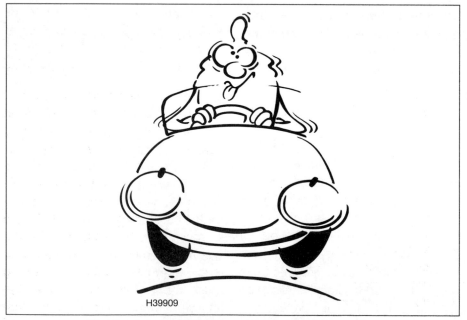

H39909

Vibration from travelling in a car can produce an erection

Dear Doctor

I am a sixteen year old male and recently I have started taking up weight training during which I have experienced something rather peculiar and unexpected. When I do the leg curl (lying face down on my weight lifting bench) after a minute or so I start to feel like I'm having an orgasm! Sometimes it feels so good I feel like I'm about to have an ejaculation. It's like another form of masturbating. Is this normal, or am I just lucky.

Forming such a meaningful and close relationship with your lifting bench is indeed lucky. All you are experiencing is a mixture of friction (it doesn't work if you lie on your back) and a poorly understood phenomenon where physical exercise translates into sexual pleasure. Watch out for photographers who have a predilection for hanging around gyms, particularly if you have any royal blood in you.

enhanced by the poorly understood phenomenon where physical exercise translates into sexual pleasure. Endorphin release from the brain may be involved. Sitting on a tumble drier, a bus, a washing machine and on people have all been reported as having the same effect.

7 Sleep

1 Sexual activity stimulates the release of endorphins from the brain. These hormones are responsible for the sensation of pleasure. Once the climax occurs blood pressure, heart rate, adrenaline release and awareness all return to, or even below, normal levels. Sleep is therefore a natural follow-up to the orgasm and many people find that masturbation is one way of getting off to sleep. You very rarely see this given as a technique for the treatment of insomnia but it works for a whole lot of people.

2 A recent report showed that snoring during pregnancy may be harmful. For many men doing the same during conception can be pretty life threatening too. One answer is more foreplay, to allow the partner to have their pleasure as well. Falling asleep together can then be fun and loving.

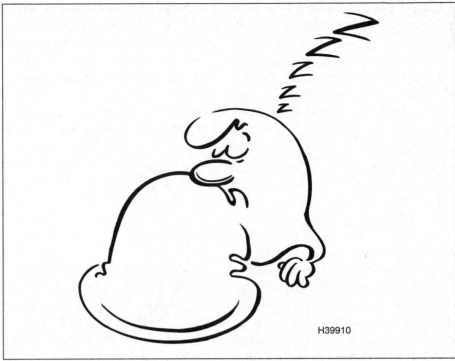

Sleep is a natural follow up to the orgasm

Dear Doctor

I am a 24 year old male and have a problem which I think is pretty common. Whenever I've had sex previously or when I make love to my girlfriend, after I have an orgasm I can't help but fall asleep. Whether it's me rolling off her, or her on top, within seconds I'm completely shattered and have gone to sleep. This has hurt the feelings of anyone I have done the deed with, because they always want for us to kiss and cuddle, hold each other, etc. I have tried all manner of things to prevent myself from nodding off – for example, splashing cold water on my face and holding my eyes open. Although a comical problem, I still would very much appreciate your help to keep me awake, and welcome any suggestions to solve this embarrassing problem.

You may not know that you become responsive to stimulation again fairly soon after the climax, unless it is late at night and you go into your normal sleep pattern. Ask your girlfriend to wake you through playing with you in whatever way comes to mind. You might not wake up but I'll bet your dreams will be pretty interesting.

8 Sex and disability

1 While a recent study showed that GPs ask about a person's sex life at the end of most consultations, disabled people are hardly ever asked at all! Recognition of the sexual needs and frustrations of disabled people received a boost with the formation of SPOD, an association with the aim of aiding the sexual and personal relationships of people with a disability. For a long time it was considered reasonable that disabled women and men should not have the same sexual

5

desires as the able-bodied variety. The irony is that much of the romantic and erotic literature is written by disabled people. An even greater irony is that many of the positions for sex and masturbation cited in the Kama Sutra, for instance, are utilised by disabled people for making love. Truly there is nothing new under the sun when it comes to sex.

2   Many people with disabilities find that sexual intercourse in the traditional position (ie, missionary – man on top, woman on her back, face-to-face for heterosexuals) is often difficult, sometimes painful, or just plain impossible. A change to some other position can often help to solve this problem. Unfortunately, other positions are often considered to be kinky or abnormal. It is important to recognise that no position for sex is abnormal or kinky. What is needed however, is a sense of humour. And a degree of patience. It may take a little time, and trial and error, to find a new position which is comfortable and satisfying for both partners but it will usually be worth it in the end.

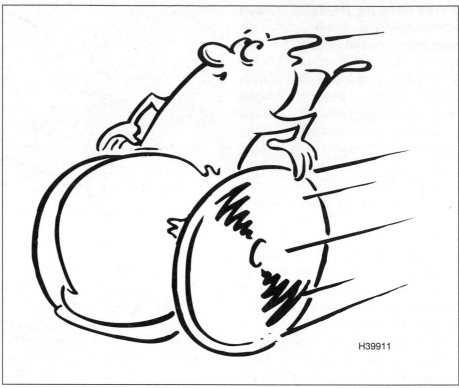

H39911

Much of the romantic and erotic literature is written by disabled people

9   Lateral thinking

1   Forget about convention and the 'missionary' position. There is no good reason why the woman should not go on top, either lying on the man or straddling his hips in a kneeling or lying position. This is particularly true for older people who may have arthritis. Don't fall into the familiarity trap, where you can only make love in a certain way because 'that's the way you do it'. You don't always need to lie down, intercourse is possible in various ways with either or both partners standing, kneeling, crouching or sitting down. It is for this reason that you may have found yourself in a tall building waiting for a lift which never seems to arrive only to discharge two slightly sweaty people when it does.

Dear Doctor

I am disabled from cerebral palsy. As it happens I did not suffer from sexual frustration until I was eighteen. Then I realised that I was missing out on more than just freedom of movement and expression. Masturbation has been difficult. Most of the time I just rub myself against the bed. It works but is not very satisfactory. I have used vibrators but it can be even more frustrating trying to attach them and switch them on. My dream was to meet someone who would understand. My dream came true when I met my partner. Unfortunately we are both disabled and find it difficult to use the 'normal' methods so we've invented a few of our own. I've heard of SPOD but never contacted them. Do you think it would help?

SPOD (the Association to Aid the Personal and Sexual Relationships of People with a Disability) used to be an excellent source of advice to help disabled people enjoy sex. Unfortunately at the time of writing the organisation was no longer functioning, although the web site forum was still in use (www.spod-uk.org).

2 The following positions are well worth considering by both the disabled and able-bodied.

- In the lying position, the woman lies on her front, with her buttocks slightly raised, while the man lies on top of her or supports his weight on his elbows and knees.
- Both may stand, the woman bending forward, preferably with some support.
- If a disability allows, a number of kneeling and crouching positions can be used.
- The rear entry position might be useful for a woman who is unable to bend her hips or knees.
- If both partners are fairly slim, they can lie on their sides, either facing each other or with the man behind the woman.
- In some of these positions, one partner may lie on a pillow to make up for their difference in breadth of hip.

Grasping the flesh

3 Achieving any contact between the important bits of the individual partners' bodies creates difficulties. More to the point some bits frankly get in the way. Getting around the problem may take some lateral thinking.

- For example, the woman may lie across a bed (or washing machine/television/pool-table) with her buttocks resting on its edge and her legs clear of support while the man enters her from any position which they find suitable. Jumping off the wardrobe is an optional extra.
- Given a little practice, sex can also take place in a sitting position. The man sits with his partner straddling his legs, facing toward or away from him. This may require more movement by the woman, although the man may assist by placing his hands around or below her buttocks.
- You can reverse the position, with the woman sitting in an armchair, with her legs drawn up as far as possible. The man can then enter her from a suitable position. The big plus is the woman in this position does not have prolonged pressure on any of her joints. A woman who is unable to bend her hips and/or straighten her knees might find this position comfortable.

4 As in any relationship, shyness can often prevent couples from openly and freely discussing topics such as alternative positions. Instead of wishing your partner has the power of mind reading, tell them what you would love to happen.

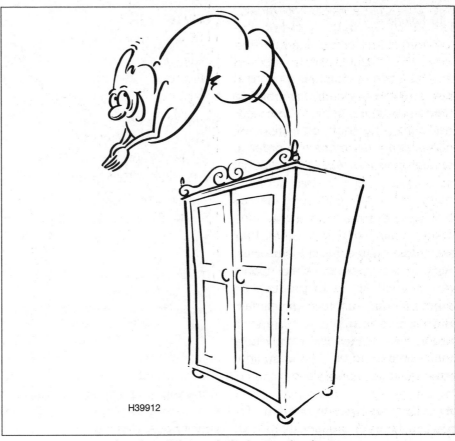

Jumping off the wardrobe is an optional extra

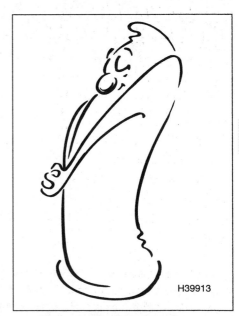

Shyness can often prevent open discussions

5

10 Faking it

1 There is a tremendous amount of pressure on both women and men to 'perform' when it comes to sex. It is not surprising that some men will actually fake an orgasm in order to appear more sexually charged. What is surprising is that this happens quite often amongst young men as well as older men. For some men faking a climax is necessary if they are not going to exhaust themselves. Alcohol has a profound effect upon a man's ability both to produce an erection and achieve a climax. Rather than admit to 'brewer's droop', some men will simply fake their climax and usually go straight into thankful, if noisy, sleep.

2 It is actually more common for men to fake an orgasm than most women realise. Because of the emphasis we put on reaching a climax some men feel they are

Dear Doctor

I am in my 60th year and have had a very good sex life with my wife for many years. However, of late, I have had difficulty in reaching a climax even though I have very little problem in achieving an erection. My penis does not seem to have the same sensitivity and I have great difficulty in ejaculating, in some cases there is very little or no ejaculation of fluid, and I feel that I am drying up. By the time I have reached a climax I am absolutely exhausted. Twice recently I've had to fake a climax (I thought only women did this) to avoid complete exhaustion and loss of erection. Is this the start of the end of my love life? Could this be prostate trouble and should I seek help from my GP?

Tiredness, alcohol abuse, anxiety and predictability are all possible causes of the problem. It is unlikely that there is any medical problem, but if you have some reason to be concerned about your prostate you should see your doctor.

failures if they do not achieve one. The production of semen is fairly constant and limited so you can temporarily deplete your stores by multiple ejaculations.

3 Tiredness, anxiety and familiarity can also be causes of the problem.

As time goes by, sexual play can become so familiar that it becomes predictable. It would be a good idea to introduce some excitement and variation. The use of erotic literature and videos can have a dramatic effect upon some people's jaded sex lives.

Chapter 6
Bodily functions

Contents

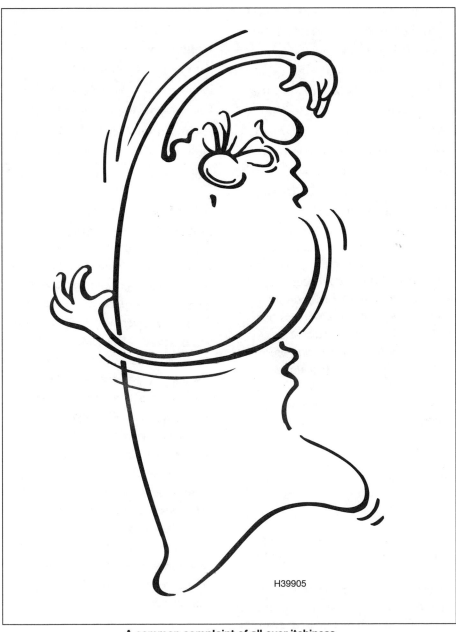

A common complaint of all over itchiness

1 Allergies

1 Being allergic to the one you love sounds like science fiction. Yet some people claim to have some sort of reaction to their partner. How this squares up with evolution is difficult to imagine as the human race would have died out years ago. There could be a simple answer however. Soap and body sprays are a common cause. When sex is anticipated a lorry load of deodorant, soap, aftershave and perfume gets dumped in those regions with natural smells completely different to Chanel No 5. It is not surprising that some reaction will take place in some people. Soap is a particular irritant but many deodorants and perfume have their own vehicles in which the active ingredients are mixed. Most aftershaves contain alcohol as an astringent which tightens the skin. Getting any of these things in your eyes gives you some idea of what they will do to the body parts which are already red.

2 A common complaint of all-over itchiness with a fine red rash is almost always a simple heat rash. Salt-laden sweat causes an intense itch which can be stopped with a quick shower, although this can raise eyebrows on an aeroplane.

6

Dear Doctor

I am 23 years old, and after making love with my girlfriend I come out in a rash which covers my whole body and it itches like mad. This stops me from giving loving kisses in the aftermath of our love making. It has never happened with any other girlfriend. Could it be to do with the fact that I do a lot of exercise?

It sounds as though you need the exercise. The rash you describe is almost certainly a simple heat rash which would respond well to showering, or in the last resort anti-histamine tablets.

3 Many couples have no problem when using a condom, but complain of pain and a rash otherwise. There are undoubtedly cases of allergy to sperm, and it may be part of the normal response to foreign bodies. Unless the woman has some reaction to sperm, pregnancy may be difficult to achieve. More often, though, the problem is not due to a reaction to the semen but rather the occupation of one partner. Farmers for instance use highly irritant chemicals which, despite protective clothing, tend to get to places they shouldn't. Even thorough washing before making love may not be enough, as it takes only traces of these chemicals to cause a reaction in such sensitive areas. Preventing the substances getting on the penis in the first place makes good sense, so adequate protective clothing is essential. Some of these chemicals are also linked with cancer so it is worth checking out. Similarly for petrol pump attendants, plasterers and woodworkers.

Dear Doctor

My boyfriend and I decided one year into our relationship that we wanted to spend the rest of our lives together. So, we decided to make love for the first time. It was so marvellous, we even came together and now we make love all the time. At first we used the Pill and condoms together, but one night we used just the Pill and I felt a painful stinging when he ejaculated inside me. I had to have a cold shower and direct the spray inside me to cool the burning sensation down. The next day a red rash appeared. We have been to a clinic and neither of us have any infections. Am I allergic to my boyfriend's sperm?

Such a shame. A truly romantic story ruined. It is interesting that you chose to use both the oral contraceptive pill and condoms. The Pill will prevent you from unwanted pregnancies but not sexually transmitted diseases. Condoms provide protection from both. It was only when you stopped using condoms your problems started. The answer could lie in your boyfriend's occupation.

2 Breasts

1 For many women all their problems would be solved if only they just had bigger breasts. At the same time an equal number of women wish they had smaller breasts. Media pressure through fashion has a lot to answer for.

Dear Doctor

I have decided to have a breast enlargement but since my consultations I have been very confused. One doctor says that oil implants are better than silicone but another doctor I consulted said that silicone implants guarantee a much better result. In America, he told me, women who have the oil ones have to sign a form saying that they cannot sue if things go wrong because oil implants are not approved by the government. Please help me to understand which is better – oil or silicone. Which doctor shall I trust?

Silicone implants have received a bad press because of leakage. Manufacturers are being taken to court by women who claim to be ill or in some way damaged because of the silicone. It is a rubbery, semi-liquid substance which was thought to be inert. Unfortunately some women have had quite serious reactions to the material which is difficult to remove once it has moved throughout the body. Soya oil is used for some implants. It works well but unfortunately can be disastrous in women allergic to soya. Water is also used although some women complain of a swishing noise when they move. Air balloons are not used. Not only would they expand in aircraft which pressurise lower than sea level pressure, a leak could be lethal causing an embolus.

The 'ideal' breasts have gone from voluptuous (Marilyn Monroe) to non-existent (Twiggy) and back again (Pamela and Jordan). Before contemplating any surgery there should be counselling. This comes before any treatment by reputable plastic surgeons. Tragically some women have breast surgery only to find they are just as unhappy afterwards.

Inverted nipples

2 Inverted nipples are common. If they have been that way for a long time there is unlikely to be any problem. If it has only happened over the past year or so a doctor should be consulted, particularly if there are any lumps or discharges. Breast cancer can show itself in this way. It is possible to bring the nipple back out into the correct position using plastic surgery. This may be available through the NHS.

3 Cystitis

1 Women suffer most from this infection of the bladder which makes them pass water more often, sometimes with a burning sensation. Men appear to get off lightly because of the greater distance between the anus, from where most of the bacteria come, and the urethra through which urine is passed.

Symptoms

- Burning sensation when passing water.
- A feeling of needing to pass water very often.

Causes

2 The most common cause is bacterial infection from the anus. It also appears to happen spontaneously, with some people suffering more than others. Diabetes and the use of steroids for chronic conditions like rheumatoid arthritis tend to make infection more common. Kidney stones and reflux (where the urine can pass back from the bladder toward the kidney) can also increase the frequency of infection.

Prevention

3 Drinking plenty of fluids helps prevent cystitis in the first place, cranberry juice which is slightly acidic is said to help prevent and treat cystitis.

Complications

4 Generally cystitis is not dangerous, but advice should be sought if there are repeated infections, because they may be due to some underlying condition such as diabetes or reflux which can damage the kidneys over a long period of time.

Self care

- Put a covered hot water bottle against the tummy to ease the pain.
- Drink slightly acid drinks such as cranberry juice, lemon squash or pure orange juice.
- Try a mixture of potassium citrate, available from your pharmacist.

See your doctor

- If symptoms persist for more than one day, or there is a fever.
- If there is any blood in the urine.
- If the sufferer is pregnant.

5 Take a urine sample from the first visit to the toilet in the morning. Use a clean, well-rinsed bottle.

4 Endometriosis

1 For centuries women have reported bleeding during their periods from places like the nose. Difficult to explain until the structure of the womb was worked out. The lining of the womb (uterus) is called the endometrium. Each month this layer of cells grows in size, then is shed with the period. These cells should normally only be found lining the womb but in some cases they migrate to different parts of the body, usually the inside of the abdomen. They still respond to the hormonal changes which take place every month and will bleed despite being in the wrong place. This produces cysts around the area. More rarely they lodge in other parts of the body.

Symptoms

2 Most women will not be aware of endometriosis as thankfully most of these cells will not cause any major problems, but they can cause severe abdominal or back pain which gradually gets worse as each period approaches. There may be heavy periods with large amounts of blood loss so anaemia can be a problem. Sexual intercourse can also be painful, especially near the time of a period.

Causes

3 The endometrial cells will only cause these problems before the menopause. They shrivel away without the promoting influence of female hormones, so it is more common between the ages of 30 and 40 years.

Prevention

4 Although the reason remains obscure, having children appears to reduce the risk of endometriosis.

6

Complications

5 The commonest complication is simply pain, but reduced fertility, ectopic pregnancy and depression may result from severe endometriosis.

Treatment

6 Herbal treatments are advocated by some. Hormones, given by mouth, injection, nasal spray or skin patch, may help reduce the activity of the endometrial cells until menopause. In severe cases surgery using laser or electrocautery can reduce the symptoms of endometriosis by removing the bulk of the cells.

5 Fibroids

1 Lots of myths surround fibroids. They are not a result of promiscuity, alcohol abuse or pregnancies that did not go through to completion. These growths are benign tumours of the womb and are not malignant. They form either within the wall of the uterus (womb), on the outside or inside the womb itself. Their size varies from pea sized to golf ball, as does the speed with which they grow. Although most common in women around 45 years old, around 20% of women aged 30 years or over will have fibroids.

Symptoms

2 Most women are completely unaware of fibroids, especially if they are only pea sized. For some women however they can cause prolonged, heavy and painful periods. In rare cases a fibroid can be felt as a hard lump in the lower abdomen, which if it presses on the bladder may cause pain on passing water or sexual intercourse.

Causes

3 The cause of fibroids is not known, but for some reason they are more common in Afro-Caribbean women.

Prevention

4 There is no known way to prevent fibroids; it used to be thought that early pregnancy reduced the risk.

Complications

5 Fibroids were often removed unnecessarily, but actually they only rarely cause pain from a lack of blood supply, requiring an operation to remove them. If they grow large enough they can prevent conception and even cause miscarriage. The good news is that fibroids tend to decrease in size after the menopause.

6 Hormone Replacement Therapy (HRT)

1 In the Western world the average woman now lives for about 30 years after the menopause. After the menopause women are liable to progressive loss of bone strength (osteoporosis) and an increasing risk of heart attacks and strokes. Studies have shown that post-menopausal women taking HRT have marked physical and other advantages over those not taking HRT.

2 Less certain than its role in preventing osteoporosis is the claim for preventing coronary heart disease. HRT is often mentioned in connection with the common menopausal symptoms such as hot flushes, night sweats, mood swings and depression. These are very

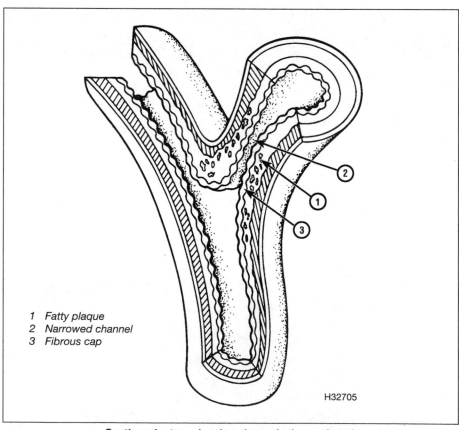

1 Fatty plaque
2 Narrowed channel
3 Fibrous cap

H32705

Section of artery showing signs of atherosclerosis

unpleasant but they are not likely to continue for very long and there is no very clear medical evidence that these symptoms are necessarily due to oestrogen deficiency. Oestrogens are, however, widely prescribed for them and many people are convinced that they help.

3 The three really important problems affecting a high proportion of post-menopausal women are loss of bone strength; the rising risk of the arterial disease atherosclerosis; and vaginal dryness and shrinkage with a resulting increase in urinary infections. Loss of sex drive may also be a problem.

Definite advantages of HRT

4 After the menopause, 3 to 5 per cent of the mass of bone is lost every year because of the lack of oestrogen. (The pre-menopause rate after age 40 is 0.3 to 0.5 per cent per year.) Ten or 20 years after menopause, a woman's bones may be brittle and can break easily after a fall, with serious results. This is one of the main reasons for hip replacement and hip repair.

5 As result, the incidence of bone fractures on minor trauma rises steeply with increasing age. Spinal column fractures, spinal curvature from bone softening, hip fractures and forearm fractures become extremely common. Osteoporosis causes fractures on minimal exposure to damage in at least a quarter of elderly women. These fractures often have serious consequences.

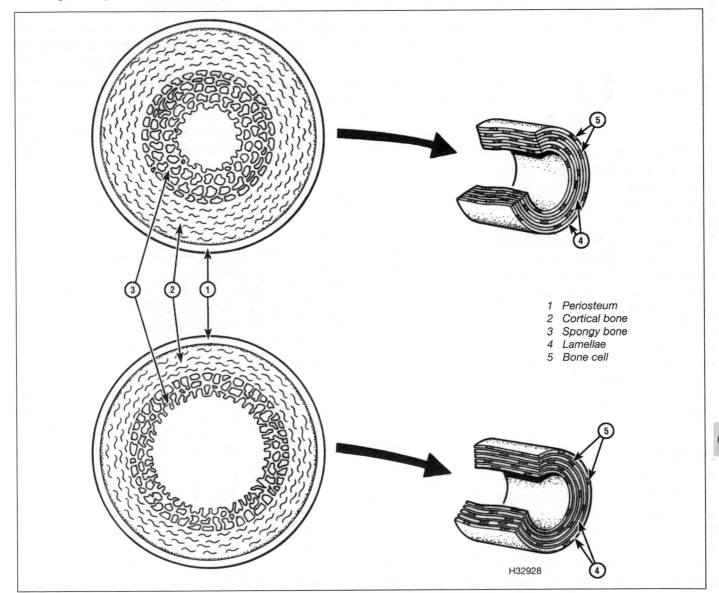

1 Periosteum
2 Cortical bone
3 Spongy bone
4 Lamellae
5 Bone cell

H32928

Normal (top) and osteoporitic bone

6 Women generally have a much lower risk of heart disease and stroke before menopause than men do. After the menopause, this risk soon rises to almost equal the risk in men. Most women think that breast cancer is their biggest killer in older age, not so. Women die more commonly from heart disease. Earlier trials suggested that women on HRT have about half the risk of coronary heart disease of those not on it. There is also the undeniable fact that HRT reduces the levels of the dangerous blood cholesterol carriers (low-density lipoproteins) by 10 to 14 per cent, and raises the levels of safe cholesterol carriers (high-density lipoprotein) by 7 to 8 per cent. These changes are known to be associated with a reduced risk of atherosclerosis and heart attacks.

7 What we know is that HRT does not affect the progression of established atherosclerosis or coronary heart disease, nor does it reduce the death rate in women who already have coronary heart disease. There is also some evidence that HRT does not, in fact, reduce heart attacks and strokes in women with no pre-existing disease.

Sandy bits

8 On the big plus side, there are few doubts about the value of local oestrogens in preventing and even treating post-menopausal vaginal dryness and atrophy (shrinkage). It is, of course, a major cause of post-menopausal sexual difficulty and will often make sexual intercourse virtually impossible, with visions of sandpaper meeting sandpaper.

9 The vaginal skin depends on oestrogen for the health, thickness and lubrication of its surface layer. Oestrogen lack causes it to thin and become dry. After the menopause there is also a change in the kind of bacteria normally found in the vagina and a change in the vaginal acidity. Live natural yoghurt (applied not eaten) helps restore this balance while lubricants can reduce the need for walking like John Wayne.

10 Post-menopausal vaginal atrophy is also linked to urinary tract symptoms such as having to go to the toilet more often (frequency, urgency and incontinence) which may often be due to oestrogen deficiency rather than urinary infection. Many doctors routinely prescribe oestrogen-containing vaginal creams, pessaries or rings to treat post-menopausal vaginal atrophy.

Now the bad news

- Women on HRT with oestrogen alone have a small but definite increase in the risk of cancer of the lining of the womb (endometrial cancer). The increase is 8 to 10 times in women who use oestrogen-only HRT for 10 years or more. The effect of this is that for every 10,000 women, there will be an additional 46 cases of endometrial cancer each year.
- HRT increases the risk of deep vein thrombosis and embolism by a factor of 2 to 3.5. This applies whether oestrogen alone or the combined therapy is taken. The effect of this increase is that for every 10,000 women on HRT there will be 2 additional cases per year when compared with the same number of women not on HRT.
- There has recently been much media interest over possible links between HRT and breast cancer. Current evidence, based on trials involving over one million women, suggests that there is indeed a significant increase in the risk of breast cancer in women taking HRT. The risk is less with oestrogen-only HRT than with combined oestrogen progesterone treatments. The risk appears to reduce to normal once HRT is discontinued. For more details see www.millionwomenstudy.org.uk

The decision

11 At the end of the day, and it usually is by the time you get to see your GP, only the person concerned can make the final decision, based on good advice.

12 However, HRT really should not be taken by a woman who:

- Has unusual vaginal bleeding that hasn't been investigated.
- Has had breast or womb cancer, as dormant traces of the disease could theoretically be stimulated by HRT.
- Has had a stroke or deep vein thrombosis, or has high blood pressure.
- Has severe liver or gall bladder disease.
- May possibly be pregnant (still the most common reason for periods to stop, and a possibility for up to two years after the start of the menopause).

Treatment options

13 Because of the danger from womb cancer, oestrogen is taken alone (without progesterone), and continuously, only by women whose womb has been removed by hysterectomy.

14 Progesterone is given with oestrogen to women with a womb, as oestrogen alone could raise the risk of cancer of the lining of the womb (endometrial carcinoma). It can be given for 14 days a month (cyclical therapy), which results in a light period each month after it is stopped.

15 Combined preparations are now available that give a period only every three months. Truly continuous preparations are recommended only for women who have not had a period for a year; they produce no periods.

16 HRT can be given as daily tablets; in skin patches; as a rub-in gel; and as a pellet implanted under the skin every six months. Local oestrogen therapy for vaginal action only can be given as a vaginal pessary, cream, or ring. HRT does not suit everyone and if several different types of HRT have been tried, with side effects causing more problems than the menopause did, then it is better to stop. Some women are also allergic to the skin patches.

7 Menopause

1 Like pregnancy, the menopause it is a natural part of life and not a sign of illness. Some doctors need to be reminded of this from time to time. As the number of eggs released from the ovaries declines so the periods become irregular, shorter and eventually cease. There is no 'normal' age for this to happen and can range from 40 years to 58 years. The average age for the menopause is around 51 years. A quarter of women will experience no difference except the lack of periods, half will report mild changes and a further quarter will experience marked changes in the way they feel along with physical differences.

Symptoms

2 Few changes in life come with such variation in impact. Not all women will experience physical symptoms and their severity will also vary. Even the duration will range from a few months to a few years but the most common are:

- Hot flushes.
- Vaginal dryness.
- Pain on intercourse (mainly due to dryness).
- Sweating.
- Headaches.
- Irregular heart beats.
- Joint pain.

3 As with physical symptoms, the non physical changes also vary greatly between women but include:

- Irritability.
- Depression.
- Tiredness.
- Poor concentration.

4 These can all lead to a lack of confidence, worries over the future, poor sleep patterns and strains on relationships.

Causes

5 As said earlier the menopause is normal but that doesn't mean we can't make life better. The changes in hormonal states, particularly the drop in oestrogen levels, are the biggest factors.

Prevention

6 As menopause has been around as long as women have it is not surprising there are 'natural' treatments such as plant phyto-oestrogens which are said to act in a similar way to hormone replacement therapy (HRT). Otherwise, talk to your doctor about the pros and cons of HRT (see above).

Complications

7 The most important medical complication is osteoporosis, or bone thinning. Any vaginal bleeding, no matter how small, should be reported to the doctor if it occurs after the menopause has settled, as cancer of the womb can occur even after menopause.

Self care

8 Regular activity is valuable in maintaining muscle tone and beating depression. Any activity such as brisk walking or cycling which produces slight breathlessness is good. Even 15 minutes per day will make a big difference.

9 Vaginal lubricants will improve love making, but remember to use water-based lubricants if you or your partner are using condoms.

10 Continue to use contraception for 2 years after the last period if it ended at under 50 years old. Otherwise use contraception for 1 year.

11 Hot flushes may be found to be triggered by certain drinks. Night sweats thankfully decline, but a change of tops and nightwear at hand can help.

12 Menopause no longer makes pregnancy an impossibility. There are medical treatments which can allow a normal pregnancy for women in their 60s and onwards. The raging debate over this seems to ignore the common phenomenon of older men having children late in life.

6

8 Period pain (dysmenorrhoea)

1 Although many women suffer from period pain, its severity can vary enormously between women from very mild to severe. The pain may also vary between monthly cycles. The good news is that generally speaking, it gets better with age and after pregnancy.

Symptoms

- Cramping abdominal pains.
- Backache.
- General fatigue.
- Nausea and vomiting.
- Diarrhoea.
- Headaches.
- Pre-menstrual bloating (water retention).

Causes

2 Period pain is not just a simple nuisance, as there are two types of period pain (dysmenorrhoea):

Primary

- This usually occurs in girls/women who have just begun to menstruate. It may disappear or become less severe after a woman leaves teenage or gives birth. The cause of these menstrual cramps is thought to be related to hormone-like substances called prostaglandins. These are chemicals that occur naturally in the body. Prostaglandins can cause muscles in the uterus to go into spasm.

Secondary

- Period pain that is due to other disorders of the reproductive system, such as fibroids, endometriosis, ovarian cysts and, rarely, cancer. An intrauterine device (IUD) can also cause period pain.

Prevention

3 The oral contraceptive pill can reduce period pain dramatically. There is a version which is not used as a contraceptive, in which case you need to use other forms of contraception. Recognising when the pains are about to start (see PMS) can give you chance to start medication early thus reducing the severity of the pain.

Complications

4 Obviously uncomplicated period pain is a normal part of the female reproductive cycle, but that does not mean that it has to be suffered. If there is an underlying condition which is making things worse there is a need for medical attention.

Self care

- Anti-inflammatory drugs (including aspirin) relieve pain and inhibit the release of prostaglandins, the hormones known to trigger the pain. Paracetamol will help with pain, but will not inhibit the release of prostaglandins.
- Hot drinks do help.
- Lying on the back, knees supported with a pillow, eases the pain.
- Hot-water bottles or a hot partner help when placed on the back or abdomen so long as there is not too much pressure.
- Warm baths are better than showers.
- Gentle massage of the lower abdomen can work wonders.
- Exercise improves blood flow and may reduce period pain. A brisk walk might help.

Ring your GP/NHS Direct

- If there is period pain unlike any other time and it is getting worse.
- If there is any abnormal vaginal discharge along with the pain.
- If the pain is arriving sooner and taking longer to depart.
- If the pain is occurring in between periods as well.

9 Pre-menstrual problems (PMS)

1 Women were once advised to refrain from driving and riding horses during the pre-menstrual period. It has even been used successfully as a defence in court. In truth, not all women suffer from pre-menstrual syndrome (PMS) but for those that do, and up to 40 per cent of women still menstruating will, it can be a distressing time of the month. The severity of the syndrome varies between women and even from month to month. It is also known as pre-menstrual tension (PMT).

Symptoms

2 The most common symptoms are:

- Depression without apparent cause.
- Irritability and anxiety.
- Tiredness.
- Tender breasts.
- Headache.
- Water retention.
- Paranoia (feelings of hostility and anger).
- Desire for certain foods.

Causes

3 It is normal and hormone changes are probably a factor. Women on the oral contraceptive pill, for instance, often report a reduction in symptoms. What value it has in evolution is unclear. The level of steroid hormones affects water retention and many women report an increase in weight along with 'bloating'. There is no standard level of PMS as it varies considerably in severity between women.

Self care

- Avoid caffeine-containing drinks. Remember tea contains as much as coffee.
- Eat lightly more often.
- Reduce salt intake.
- Increasing activity levels may help.

4 As with many states of mind, PMS can be confused with depression. See your doctor if the feeling of depression never really lifts, you are waking early with poor sleep patterns or if you feel like hurting yourself or someone else.

10 Testosterone Replacement Therapy (TRT)

1 Despite controversy, HRT for women has a lot going for it. Although early claims proved to be too optimistic, HRT for women has a place in the prevention of osteoporosis – thinning of the bones. In the USA a patch has been developed which gradually releases testosterone, the male sex hormone. It is now available in the UK. There have been enthusiastic reports in the media over the effects this can have on libido, muscle development and general well-being. Unfortunately most of the information comes from an ill-informed press. When things are not going quite right in the sex department, at work or within the

family, it is tempting to look for a simple reason. Lack of testosterone, the male sex hormone, is an easy target. Hormone Replacement Therapy (HRT) for men, or more accurately Testosterone Replacement Therapy (TRT), has become a real possibility.

Role of testosterone

2 Testosterone is released from the testes under direct control of a small gland in the brain called the pituitary. It secretes FSH (follicle stimulating hormone) which stimulates the production of sperm and LH (leutenising hormone) which stimulates the testes to produce testosterone. It is partly responsible for secondary male characteristics such as facial hair. It also has a role in maintaining muscle power and keeps your tackle in good order.

Blood levels of testosterone remain fairly steady with a gradual fall over the years. Testosterone exerts a diminishing effect as we get older, not least because the hormone is increasingly 'capped' by a protein which prevents it from stimulating body function (think of a sword inside a scabbard), but big drops in blood levels only occur with damage or disease of either the pituitary or testes. Men with hypogonadism have a reduction in the amount of testosterone in their blood. Hormone replacement for these men is essential to maintain normal body functions. This is the main reason for the manufacture of testosterone hormone replacement.

Penile erectile dysfunction

3 Many men who request hormone replacement therapy do so in the

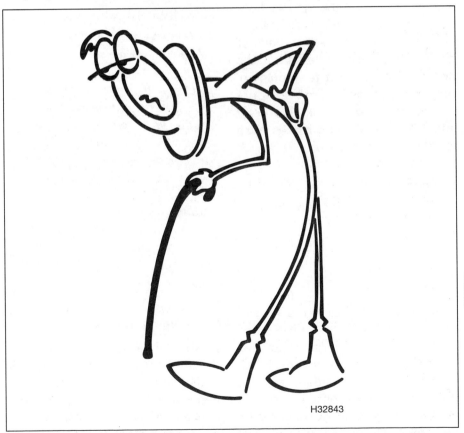

H32843

There have been reports over the effects TRT can have on libido, muscle development and general well-being

6

hope of correcting their penile erectile dysfunction, or impotence. Such problems are common, but a low level of testosterone is less often the cause than say diabetes, high blood pressure, atherosclerosis or the drugs they are taking either as prescription medicines or in the form of alcohol (see *Erectile dysfunction*). Levels of testosterone are usually normal in men with erectile dysfunction. Sexual problems, stress, tiredness or marital disharmony are also more commonly the main culprits.

Building hormone

4 Testosterone's involvement in building muscles has been exploited by men obsessed with body building. Earlier forms of testosterone were dangerous in high doses and have been withdrawn in the UK. Even so, although injections of high doses of testosterone increase muscle mass they can still have serious side effects on the heart and liver. Short-term gains of bulging muscles are a poor recompense for a weakened heart and a failing liver. It only makes you a healthy-looking corpse.

Danger

5 Some cancers are stimulated to grow by hormones. Prostate cancer, which kills over 9,000 men in the UK each year, thrives on hydroxy-testosterone. In fact, by stopping the body producing this form of testosterone, the tumour's growth often slows down. One of the drugs used for treating enlarged prostates, finesteride (Proscar) which blocks the conversion of testosterone into the active hydroxy form, is reported as reducing prostate cancer by 25 per cent. Obviously giving high doses of testosterone to a man with

undiagnosed prostate cancer could be disastrous so they must first be carefully checked. Rectal examination with a gloved finger by your doctor gives some indication of any problems but blood tests are more accurate. Prostate specific antigen (PSA), for instance, is a good marker of prostate cancer. Unfortunately its value decreases as you get older as the levels rise even without the presence of any tumour. Ultrasound can also be useful although most doctors will require blood tests before giving any additional testosterone.

Dear Doctor

I read in the paper that men can now get hormone replacement therapy just like us women. Is this true, and what effect does it have on his sex? I thought only women could use it as it kept your breasts in shape.

Fortunately the hormone in this case is the male hormone testosterone and not the female hormone oestrogen. Getting the two mixed up could definitely have some effect on your partner's sexual activity, but not in the way you would appreciate. Testosterone patches certainly help men who have a proven lack of their own natural hormone but the jury is still out over its use for the so called 'male menopause' if it even exists.

The male menopause

6 We do know that it is at this time of life that uncertainty, under-confidence and inability to fit the media image of a sexually powerful, competitive macho male can affect a man's self image. It is tempting to simply put this down to a lack of sex

hormone. Compounding all this is the fear of ageing. Some of the claims for testosterone therapy go beyond simply replacing what is missing and this can be eagerly accepted by men with no organic problems.

Dear Doctor

My husband reckons he is going through the male menopause. I told him that only women can have a menopause but he is adamant and says he is suffering all things that I went through when my periods stopped. I don't want to hurt his feelings by not believing him, but it's the first time I have ever heard that men can have a menopause as well as women.

At a certain stage in a man's life, usually around 45 to 55 years of age, a so called 'mid-life crisis' can occur. It has been labelled the male menopause although there is little comparison to the female version. Unlike women, there is no evidence of a dramatic drop in sex hormone levels. Even so some workers in the area have suggested that we should measure not testosterone but FSH (follicle stimulating hormone) which stimulates sperm production and LH (leutenising hormone) which stimulates the production of testosterone. Similarly, testosterone circulates in the blood attached to a protein, sex hormone binding globulin (SHBG). This can inactivate the hormone until released. The levels of bound testosterone gradually rise with age, thus reducing the effects of testosterone on the target organs. Perhaps the reason why we don't have any evidence of hormonal variation is because we are looking at the wrong hormones.

Check it out

7 Many things have an effect on testosterone levels. Chronic alcohol abuse, for instance, reduces the ability of the testes to produce testosterone. If you think you would benefit from TRT, get it clear in your mind *why* you would like it and then sit down with your doctor. Most of the problems people hope to be 'cured' by male HRT can be solved without any hormone treatment.

8 Check out the basics first:

- Sort out problems with your partner, counselling can help.
- Take a close look at your lifestyle and see if you are smoking, drinking to excess or avoiding exercise. This will all contribute to

the vicious circle of feel bad factors.

- Ditch that beer gut. Only people like Oscar Wilde got away with it anyway.
- Relax, rather than collapse. You can be active and yet relax. Kids are a marvellous source of cheap entertainment and relaxation, if you are prepared to be the horse/elephant/train.
- Despite the previous point, get rid of the kids now and again. Sex and intimacy can improve when the children are with someone else for the night. A romantic break can be as simple as telling the kids to entertain themselves for a couple of hours while you have a cuddle. Better still, take a night away once in a while and let

the in-laws benefit from all the exercise of being a horse/elephant/train for a change.

Further information

9 If you would like to know more, look in the Contacts section at the back of the book, or contact:

British Association for Sexual and Relationship Therapy
PO Box 13686
London
SW20 9ZH
www.basrt.org.uk

11 Grief

Scale of misery

1 Psychologists often refer to a scale which rates life events in terms of the stress they can cause. The death of a spouse comes at the very top. Many people will not admit that part of their feeling of loss comes from the absence of physical contact and sex. It is hard for anyone who has not gone through the experience to realise just how bad this can feel. Worse still, thoughts of sex with someone else bring a whole basket full of mixed emotions to the surface, not least guilt. It helps to recognise the pattern that happens when a partner is lost.

Just to help me sleep

2 Some people find it very difficult to break out of the vicious cycle of thinking about sex and the guilt it produces. Even masturbation can feel like a betrayal. Men and women find themselves enjoying company, lightly sprinkled with sexual attraction then suddenly feel guilty. Television with its goodly dollop of

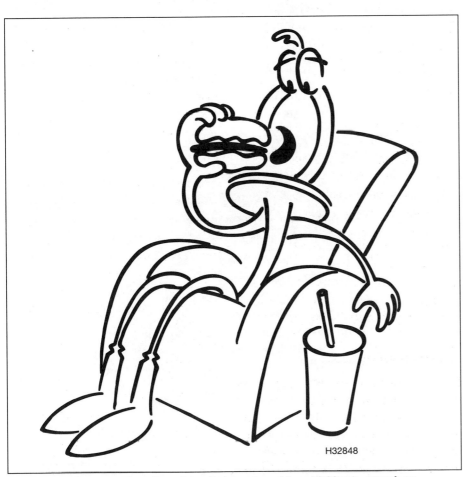

H32848

Look at your lifestyle and see if you are smoking, drinking too much or avoiding exercise

6

sexual titillation may be a form or relief but can also raise guilt feelings. Like a medical equivalent of a cold shower, many will turn to sleeping tablets. This is no surprise. The bed represents everything to do with sexual comfort and loving. Buying a different bed can be a mixture of pain and relief.

Night times

3 For most men the problems start when they wake up in the morning with an erection. The prostate holds the only known G spot for men.

Dear Doctor

I was 89 last year, and I lost my wife 3 years ago. For the last 3 months I get intense erections when waking up in the morning and have to relieve myself with a massage of soap and warm water. Is my hormone/testosterone out of order? I was sexually active since I was 14 and since then sex played a big role in my life. However, since my wife died I find it very difficult to form new relationships as all my female companions say sex is out of the question.

It sounds as though you are surfacing from your grief over losing your wife. No one will ever replace her, but there are plenty of women who would be glad of male company and sexual relationships. As men die on average six years younger than women, you are heavily outnumbered by women. Change your female acquaintances if they all feel you are too old to enjoy sex, or that you need to remain 'loyal' to your wife. You are not asking anyone to step into her shoes.

Vibration or rubbing against this gland will cause arousal. During the night your bladder fills, putting increasing pressure on the prostate. This does a very nice job of causing an erection when you wake. You may find this happens more often after a few drinks the night before. Needless to say it is normal and proves that all your tackle is in good working order. Age is no barrier to enjoying sex. Ageism, where men were dubbed 'dirty old men' if they as much as expressed any sort of sexual desire, is on the way out not least because we are all living so much longer.

Me depressed?

4 Most people underestimate the effects of bereavement on a person, until it happens to themselves. Some of these can be so bad, that the bereaved person often will not realise that the loss of interest in their job or family, constant pacing of the floor, spontaneous weeping or complete loss of appetite, are all normal and common manifestations of grieving. People who are close to the bereaved person may also become impatient with them as time wears on, again underestimating the extent of the effects, and the length of time they can be felt by the person. It is at this point that true friends are worth their weight in gold. To know when to let the person alone and when to sit and listen, often to the same story over and over again without interruption, is a gift that few people have nowadays. Bereavement can even affect the memory and people will comment upon a 'complete blank' for a period following the death. Almost every facet of life can be, and is, affected, only the scale and duration varies

Dear Doctor

I am 53 years old. My husband and only sexual partner of over 33 years, died suddenly. Marriage was not all a bed of roses. Like many couples, we had our ups and downs, but we stuck it out together, and the sexual side, in the early years, was absolutely terrific. Later on, menopause affected my needs and desires but we coped well and my husband was quite understanding. Over the past 18 months I have missed his presence and companionship, but now I'm beginning to miss the physical sexual contact and the cuddles. I am not looking for a replacement for my late husband, but any advice you can offer towards 'filling the gap' would be of great help.

Grief and grieving take their toll. Finding a replacement for your husband is impossible and undesirable. Few people will tolerate for long being compared to some former partner, and nobody will ever fill shoes that once trod paths special to you. These memories are yours and don't need to be diluted with surrogates. Look to the future. You are a young woman with a long life ahead of you. Only the most selfish of partners would wish their loved ones a life devoid of loving once they had gone forever. Look for someone different, expect different compliments, fresh observations on common scenes. There will never be anyone the same as your partner. But that's better. Cuddles from someone new, sex with a different person, is not the same as trying to pretend your partner still has you in his arms. Let the tut-tutting classes tut. Life is so very short. Look for future happiness while remembering what went before.

between people. Not being judgmental and supportive when the conversation inevitably turns to new relationships can be difficult, particularly for close relatives and children. Ageism also creeps in. Old men and women are expected to 'know their place' and not to behave in any sexually overt manner. How many poor sods have been threatened by their children with, 'What would Mummy think!' Thankfully, there are professional agencies who specialise in this form of counselling and can be contacted through your GP. Nobody pretends that strangers are as good as friends or relatives, but they can often help a person who has difficulty coming to terms with their loss.

Sex after bereavement

5   Guilt is a common emotion which often inhibits sex after a bereavement. Talking things through always helps but the patience of partners can be stretched and there is a danger of becoming 'locked in' with grief so that there is no room for anything or anyone else. There is no golden rule of thumb and people will surface at different times and have sex. Some may never recover completely and will live a celibate life thereafter. Being forced into unwilling sex is counter-productive, so gentleness and the patience of Job are great attributes. The good news is that most people do find

Dear Doctor

I am 75 years old and throughout my long marriage until my wife died I never associated with any other women except those I met on a purely friendly basis. I loved my wife very much and bitterly regret losing her so what follows is in no way derogatory. Basically, although we had regular sex throughout our marriage it was always fairly unadventurous with one main position – the missionary position. I did on one occasion suggest we find alternatives but she just didn't want to know. I accepted this but always knew that sexually things could have been considerably better between us. Recently I bought a newspaper in which women were offering sex in the guise of massage and my question to you is, do you think I could obtain from these women the kind of sex I would have enjoyed but never experienced with my wife? Certainly I would never have considered such a move whilst my wife was alive.

The relationship with your wife was very special and cannot be replaced, but it is understandable that you miss the sexual part of your relationship along with the loving that you experienced. Without doubt there are women who will be able to supply your sexual needs, but you may find it more satisfying to have a meaningful relationship with a woman which includes more than just sex. Replying to advertisements in magazines carries all the risks of exploitation on both sides, not to mention the danger of sexually transmitted diseases. Perhaps it would be better to make contact with someone new rather than take these risks.

enjoyment in sex once again, but for many there will be occasions when it will not be possible.

Points to remember

- People have different ways of expressing grief, there is no 'normal way'.
- Talk about it, even if it hurts.
- Don't be afraid to seek support from friends, relatives or your doctor.
- Aggression is natural, even towards close relatives and well meaning neighbours. Doctors are a common focus of anger.
- Allow yourself time to grieve.
- Avoid drugs, if in doubt.
- We only rent this space and life is not a dress rehearsal, this is it.

6

Chapter 7
Genital descriptions – how things work

Contents

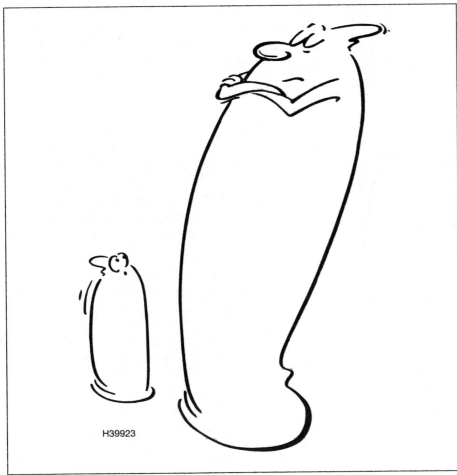

Penis size is a perennial cause of male concern

1   Penis: big is BIG

1   Penis size is a perennial cause of male concern. Most men compare themselves with the guy at the next urinal which is a mistake, not least because you may pee in his turn-ups. Looking sideways on gives an impression of length lost when looking down. It's best to use a mirror.

2   Surgery can lengthen the penis and some famous men admit to subjecting themselves and their tackle to the knife. About 50 per cent of the penis is hidden inside the pelvis, held by ligaments. These help maintain the angle of dangle during erection. By cutting these ligaments a significant increase in size can be achieved but at a cost. Instead of taking off like a Harrier jump jet it will do so like a Lancaster bomber. Losing weight can also help. Roughly one inch of penis length is gained per

7

30 pounds of excess weight lost. There is a law of diminishing returns operating here, and once you get down to a total body weight of under 7 stone you become either a jockey or a pole vaulter.

Shape

3 Men generally worry about the shape of the penis more than their nose. Most will accept a nose bent sideways at 90 degrees with little hope of disguise, yet want almost invisible kinks ironed out from their penis. The structure of the penis gives a clue to why it is the shape it is. There are two large tubes of spongy tissue, the corpora cavernosa, and a smaller tube called the corpus spongiosum. By filling these with blood the penis will enlarge, both radially and in length. If one fills less than the others, or if scarring stops one from extending as it fills, the whole thing is pulled to one side. There may well be room here for creative surgery particularly for wine lovers.

Dear Doctor

I am a 24-year-old man, with a very worrying problem. It has to do with the shape of my penis. When I become aroused, my penis grows in size and becomes hard, as normal, but it also bends quite severely downwards, so that it doesn't look like a full erection. I feel sexually inadequate because of this. I've heard of something called Peyronie's Disease. Could this be it? Also, I've read that Vitamin E might help? Is this true? I am a virgin, and because of this problem I am reluctant to form a sexual relationship with a woman. Please help.

Penises vary considerably in both size and shape. If we were to believe all the erotic or pornographic videos your penis should be at least 12 inches long and as straight as an arrow. In truth the range of size is from around three-and-a-half inches to seven inches. Most men do not have a perfectly straight penis but instead have bends in any direction. Severe angulation goes under the heading of Peyronie's disease but actually there is no single cause. We do know that trauma early on in life can produce thickened bands of tissue on one side of the penis shaft. This causes the penis to bend during erection and can make ejaculation painful. Surgery is available on the National Health Service and you should consult your general practitioner. Creams containing Vitamin E have some success in improving skin quality in the area of scars. You may try this while you are waiting for an appointment with the plastic surgeon. Meantime you might find solace in getting winkles out of their shells. It is indeed an ill wind which blows nobody any good, if we exclude winkles.

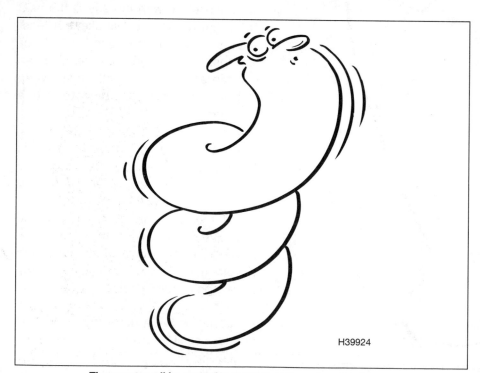

H39924

There may well be room for creative surgery for wine lovers

2 Penis injury

1 Considering the way it sticks out, you would think there would be significantly more injured penises than there are. Even so men manage to mangle, chop and burn their most prized possessions on a regular basis. Unfortunately the embarrassment factor can delay treatment. One man was cooking while naked. He had wisely put a tea towel around his chest to protect himself from fat splashing from the frying eggs. No problem. No problem, that is until he reached over to switch on the fan behind the electric cooker and his penis went under the grill. Bad enough you may

Dear Doctor

I have a real problem. When I was very young I fractured my penis (so young I don't remember how or when it happened). It makes it difficult to get close to the girls in my life to the point where I cannot stay in a relationship much beyond the first intimate contact. I am still a virgin but I want a full relationship.

Do I need surgery? If so, how much will it cost and is there any risk to the feeling in my penis?

Generally speaking, most men know when they suffered a fractured penis. Its the kind of thing that tends to stick in a person's mind. Not many of us would look down, scratch our ear and mutter, 'Now I wonder how that happened'. Physiology-wise, you can only fracture your penis while it is fully erect. The spongy tissue is then filled under pressure with blood and is extremely firm. Most injuries occur, therefore, while making love and few men would fail to notice. The penile shaft actually does break and is held together only by the skin, urethra and blood vessels. Unfortunately the blood tends to clot once blood flow becomes impossible. This makes surgery extremely difficult. With expert attention the penis can recover but tends to have bends where once there were no bends. Plastic surgery can help and it is possible to insert metal or plastic prostheses which restores an 'erection'. I suspect you never actually fractured your penis but are suffering from Peyronie's disease – see above.

say. Worse, much worse. The element was the old type with uncovered wire. Not only did he burn his penis he also experienced 230 volts in those places not designed to conduct electricity. All this only came to light when he turned up at casualty with burns to his chest from two fried eggs.

2 Energetic love making also causes casualties. Tears, fractures and even amputations occur when the red haze becomes too much, particularly if your partner has reason to believe that he or she is not the only person to have recently provided oral sex.

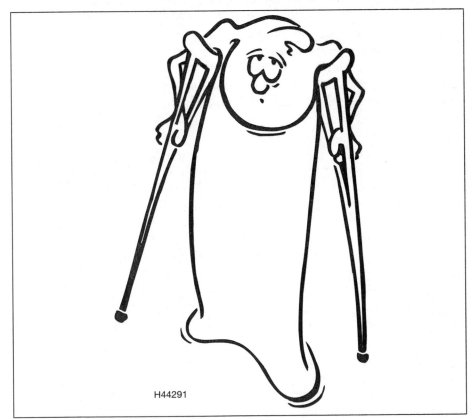

H44291

Considering the way it sticks out, you would think there would be more injured penises

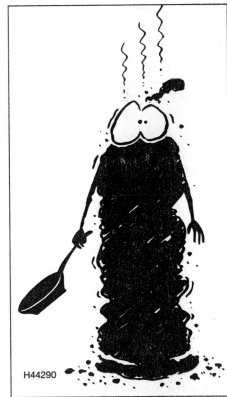

H44290

Men manage to mangle, chop and burn their most prized possessions on a regular basis

7

Dear Doctor

My problem is that when my penis is erect my foreskin remains over the helmet. When I try to pull it back it feels quite painful and I imagine that sex would also be quite painful. I have seen a couple of sex videos and all the men have their foreskin pulled back. I feel that I am abnormal in some way. Is there anything I can do about it?

Yes. Stop worrying. The foreskin sits over the helmet or glans of the penis until it is pulled back. That's why it's called a foreskin. If you haven't been pulling it back regularly during masturbation or washing then it is bound to be tight. For some men such tight pullovers can be painful when first having sex. They usually find it gets better each time, although riding a bike becomes a whole new experience for a short while. You should really be retracting your foreskin regularly anyway if only for hygiene reasons. Do it when flaccid first, then partly erect then finally, and excruciatingly, when fully erect. If it refuses to return squeeze the helmet firmly after applying an ice compress for about five minutes. It will eventually go back if you squeeze firmly enough. This takes a certain amount of courage and a goodly supply of paper tissues for your eyes. If you squeeze firmly enough for long enough the foreskin will return over the glans. Lack of success means a trip to your local casualty department, sooner rather than later.

pheromones or sex attractants. If not regularly pulled down and washed, a cheesy yellow smegma forms which reminds passing Dobermans of Grimsby fish market. You can run from a Doberman but you cannot hide. Not with four pounds of haddock down your trouser front anyway.

4 Frenulum

1 The frenulum is a thin ligament between the foreskin and the glans of the penis which can tear very easily either during masturbation or sex. It has a small artery which when cut produces a most spectacular display. Simply pressing on the bleeding point will stop it and a circumcision is rarely needed.

3 Foreskin

1 The foreskin is a thin layer of skin which normally sits over the head or glans of the penis. Its job is probably to protect the sensitive glans beneath and act as a valve along with the thickened ridge around the base of the glans preventing sperm from leaving the vagina. It has secretory glands producing substances which may act as

5 Penile bumps

1 Men and for that matter women get terribly concerned over penile bumps that appear on erection.

Dear Doctor

I have a problem of a tearing frenulum. It is a problem which I (and my wife) suffer from regularly and it is very painful. I have to stop immediately. The moment is then ruined and lost for both of us. I have been to my GP and he has prescribed a steroid cream which solves the problem for a couple of days. But what about the cause? Do I need to be circumcised? I do use a lubricant but I find that my wife does 'dry up' on me. I am 53 and my wife is 54.

I was once called out to a man who was absolutely distraught. He and his wife were having sex while she was 7 months pregnant. Suddenly blood was everywhere. He thought he had caused an abortion, which is almost totally impossible through sex during a normal pregnancy. It transpired he had torn his frenulum . Relief was not the word when I explained what had happened. Only then did he suddenly notice the pain in his penis. Regular use of powerful steroid creams are not a good idea. They can actually cause a weakening of the ligament and the surrounding skin, making it more likely to break again. You almost certainly do not need a circumcision. Once you stop using the steroid cream and use a good lubricant things should improve. I suspect your partner is anticipating another 'disaster' and this is causing her to go dry. More foreplay will also help, or try using a condom. If all else fails you can have the frenulum removed by minor surgery. Either that or find a very large pencil sharpener.

Sweat glands and hair follicles stand out on the penis when it is erect, just like goose pimples. The skin is so thin they are pushed outwards by the hard shaft immediately underneath. The only other things that could possibly be a cause of 'bumps' are warts.

Dear Doctor

They say doctors have heard it all, but have you heard this before? I love my boyfriend but I hate his willy. The ridge is covered with whitish, pimply bumps. He promised he hadn't had sex with anyone else and I believe him. The problem is I don't want to have oral sex with him. He won't go to the doctor. What are they? Can they be removed?

He probably doesn't need to see a doctor. Sweat glands and hair follicles stand out on the penis when it is erect. The only other things that could possibly be a cause are warts. Genital warts tend to be tiny but may clump together like a cauliflower. They are usually caught off someone else during intercourse but it is possible to develop warts anywhere on your body without such contact. If they are warts, they can be removed at a genito-urinary clinic. He shouldn't try to do this himself as it makes the eyes water terribly.

6 Cancer of the penis

1 Penile cancer is thankfully rare. One or two men per 100,000 will develop the cancer with approximately 100 men dying each year in the UK. It is a disease of older men, usually over 65 years of age. If caught early it is eminently treatable with a 90 per cent survival rate. Despite this, many men consult their doctor too late. Smegma may be a culprit. Circumcised men rarely develop the tumour and it is almost unheard of in men circumcised at birth. Personal hygiene is considered important for the same reason but as a justification for boyhood circumcision it is debatable given the relative rarity of the condition.

Check it out
- Carefully check the region between the glans and the foreskin.
- Look for small, often painless ulcers or warty nodules. Difficulty in retracting the foreskin, may indicate tethering at this point.
- A persistent red velvet-like patch on the glans needs medical attention even if it is painless.

Safe but scary
- Tiny bumps all over the shaft are just sweat glands. The penile skin is so thin they stand out.
- Bleeding from beneath the foreskin after vigorous sex or masturbation is common – the skin between the foreskin and the glans is easily torn. If it persists see your doctor.
- It is easy to bruise the skin in the same way with dramatic purple patches appearing the next day. They should disappear in a few days.

Treatment

2 Anti-cancer drugs can be applied as a paste to the tumour itself. Localised radiotherapy and laser surgery are also used. More advanced cases require partial amputation, a couple of centimetres back from the growth. Cosmetic surgery restores normal services in the sex and water works departments. Advanced cases involve total amputation and the days of hitting flies on the wall are gone forever. Keep an eye on what is under the fly on your trousers, or buy a swatter.

7 Circumcision

1 We have a strange, love–hate relationship with circumcision. As a society we tolerate male circumcision yet the majority of us find female circumcision abhorrent. Words such as mutilation are commonly levied at those who surgically remove a girl's clitoris, yet medical and ritualistic circumcision of boys is commonplace. As a nation the UK performs this operation for 'medical reasons' twice as often as most other European countries. Either they are performing too few circumcisions or British doctors too many. It is possible to restore the foreskin, but it takes patience and perseverance. Weights are applied to a ring which sits around the base of the glans, progressively stretching the remains of the foreskin. The process is similar to that employed by some African tribes for extending their necks, lips or tongues.

Further information

2 If you would like to know more, look in the Contacts section at the back of the book, or contact:
NORM-UK
www.norm-uk.org

7

Dear Doctor

I had a circumcision 6 months ago to rid myself of an old problem I've had for 5 years. Everything went fine and the old problem cleared up thanks to the operation. The only problem is I have been left with a very ugly scar and a ridge around my penis. It looks ugly and this is worrying me. Can you tell me if the scar will fade because it certainly doesn't look as if it will. And will the ridge surrounding the scar go down and disappear? Also, it's still very sensitive. Will this also get better with time?

Obviously I don't know what your original problem was, possibly a phimosis or tight pullover as it is called in the trade. Having your foreskin stuck in the retracted position is not good fun. One guy came into casualty unable to bear the pain after two days. His glans was the size of a small orange but quite different in colour. Circumcision is the definitive answer but is not always necessary. With any surgery some scarring is inevitable. You can try ointments containing Vitamin E which promote normal skin healing. Unfortunately once the scar is well established success is limited. Further surgery to remove the scar only increases the risk of making an even larger scar. Keloid is a type of scar tissue which resembles callus seen on trees after branches have been cut off. It is ugly and difficult to treat. Check with your GP. If your original operation was performed under the NHS you may be able to have plastic surgery to correct the problem.

8 Balanitis xerotica obliterans

1 Far from being a vaguely illegal sexual position this clinical problem can make most positions uncomfortable. Any medical condition containing the term 'xerotica' means the docs don't know and frankly must be something you did against good advice from your mother. More common than we think, this condition causes a thickening of the tissue beneath the skin making the foreskin less elastic and difficult to retract. Classically it causes 'ballooning' when passing water but more importantly makes sex very uncomfortable. It can sometimes be treated with topical steroids or daily application of Aloe Vera, but if it continues to cause problems a circumcision is on the cards.

9 Priapism

1 Now here is a nasty one. As if getting it up is not difficult enough, sometimes it is impossible to get the damn thing back where it belongs, or at least when you are talking to your girlfriend's mother. Priapism is a prolonged and painful penile erection in the absence of any sexual interest. It results from the failure of the normal return of blood from the spongy tissue (corpora cavernosa) of the penis to the circulation at the termination of a period of sexual excitement (detumescence), which is just jargon for blood being where it shouldn't be, and far too much of it as well.

2 This can be painful and eye-wateringly persistent. There are cases of men having erections for 24 hours. Sadly, this is not quite the fun it sounds.

3 Priapism may happen for a variety of reasons. In some cases there is a disturbance of the nervous control of blood flow, to and from the penis, due to disease of the spinal cord or brain. In others, blood disorders, such as leukaemia or sickle cell disease, may be causing partial clotting (coagulation) of the blood in the penis. Inflammation of the prostate gland (prostatitis) can cause this, as can a stone (calculus) in the bladder, or urethritis, which interferes with the normal outflow of blood from the penis.

4 Perhaps the most common cause though is the incorrect use of injection drugs to produce an erection. Resist the temptation to use your mate's injection system as he may suffer from diabetes and need a much higher amount of drug than you could possibly need. Failing to remove the rubber ring used in conjunction with vacuum devices can also be a problem although for most men the ring will slip off after intercourse.

5 You do need to know why this is happening as there may be an underlying condition needing your doctor's attention. Also, a long-sustained erection is dangerous because of the risk of clotting in the corpora cavernosa of the penis. Such thrombosis produces serious and permanent loss of erectile function, so treatment must be prompt and effective.

6 It is possible to reverse the effects of drugs used for producing erections by injecting the penis with

other drugs. This may also be useful for other causes of priapism. In rare cases it may be necessary to remove blood from the penis using a syringe. This is the kind of thing you really don't want to hear about let alone see. If you are having trouble reducing an erection go to the local A&E department, forget about embarrassment, you are talking serious high voices here.

10 Prostate

Fuel mixture valve problems

1 A Men's Health Forum survey in 2002 showed that men have an increasingly better awareness about their prostate. This was blemished just a tad by 10 per cent of those men surveyed saying that women also had prostates. Less than one in ten knew the risk from prostatism at some time in a man's life (50/50) and half of men thought a red rash on the penis is a sign of prostate problems (it isn't). Women scored much higher for knowledge about men's bodies as well as their own. There is no euphemism for the prostate, but if there were it would probably be a 'fuel mixture valve for the rocket'. This is not a million miles away from the truth. The prostate does act as a one-way valve preventing urine and sperm mixing, and also produces a battery of nutrients to keep sperm alive and kicking. Prostate cancer kills around 10,000 men in Britain every year, yet because it is slow growing most men will die with it rather than because of it. Men have the same risk of developing prostate cancer as women have of breast cancer. Benign prostatic hyperplasia (enlargement of the prostate) is even more common, with trans-urethral resection of prostate (TURP) being the single greatest male surgical procedure in the UK. Prostatitis is found in younger men and is basically a mystery when it comes to cause. Treatment, not surprisingly, tends to be hit and miss.

The root of the problem

2 If you have found that as time goes by you are unable to push the deodorant blocks down the channel in the urinal, relax. You are in good company. Obstruction of the flow of urine by an enlarged prostate is common, particularly as we get older. Sitting at the neck of the bladder, straddling the tube which carries urine and semen, the prostate is roughly the size of a walnut and has an important job of providing nutrients and protection for the sperm about to make the long journey to the womb. The vagina is a hostile place so far as sperm are concerned. Prostatic secretions help neutralise the acid environment found in the vagina. Sperm have little room for carrying fuel for energy. The prostate produces large amounts of

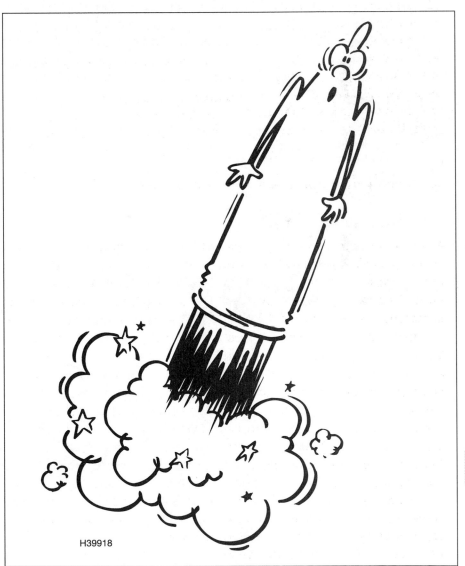

H39918

There is no euphemism for prostate, but it would probably be a 'fuel mixture valve for the rocket'

7

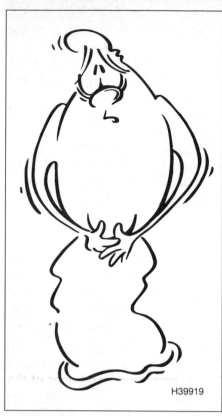

Should the prostate enlarge it can completely halt the flow of urine

fructose, an easily absorbed sugar, to keep the engines running. It has nothing to do with the sex drive, which is a shame as it enlarges with age. Should the prostate enlarge too much it can obstruct and even completely halt the flow of urine from the bladder to the penis. When this is caused by simple enlargement with no involvement of cancer, it is referred to as Benign Prostatic Hypertrophy (BPH).

Common problem

3 Over 30 per cent of men will have some problem with passing urine by the time they reach 50 years of age, yet only half of those men suffering will consult their doctor. Most men put it down to the inevitability of ageing. Many men, as high as 20 per cent of 40 year olds, will need some form of treatment before they die. We don't know why it enlarges but there are certain triggers:

- High levels of testosterone.
- An imbalance between oestrogen and testosterone.
- Possibly, low protein, high carbohydrate diets.
- Western diets.

Symptoms of an enlarged prostate

4 Sure signs of an enlarged prostate are:

- Poor flow.
- Frequent trips to the toilet, especially during the night.
- A persistent feeling of 'not quite emptying the bladder' often associated with dribbling after passing urine.
- Traces of blood in the urine or sperm sometimes occur and should always be reported to your doctor.

5 Your doctor can perform a few simple tests to check the size of your prostate and make sure it is nothing nasty.

Detection

6 The way an enlarged prostate affects you is very important to your doctor. Just from your description alone a working diagnosis can often be made. By examining your rectum with a gloved finger your doctor can check whether your prostate is enlarged. Blood tests will also give some indication of why your prostate is enlarged as some of the tests (prostate specific antigen – PSA – or acid phosphatase) are fairly specific for cancer. Ultrasound is also used by passing a sensor into the rectum to visualise the prostate.

Treatment

7 Thankfully men are not doomed to walking around with a street map

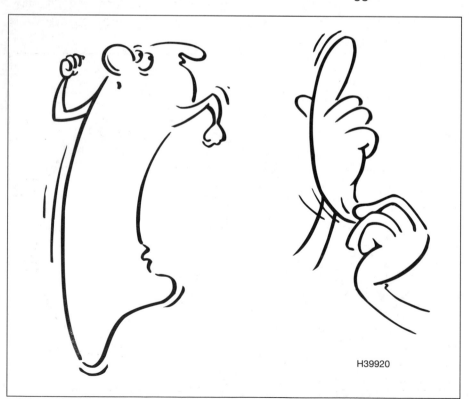

By examining your rectum with a gloved finger your doctor can check your prostate

showing all the public conveniences. There are basically two options, drugs or surgery.

Drugs

8 A number of medications are available which relax the muscles which are making matters worse. Side effects of the more commonly used versions include a dry mouth and a slow response from the heart when standing up. This might cause a drop in blood pressure and thus dizziness.

Surgery

9 If drugs fail or the obstruction becomes complete, surgery is required. What was once a major operation is now simplicity itself. Trans-urethral prostatectomy (TURP) has revolutionised the treatment of enlarged prostates. There are now 40,000 prostatectomies performed in the UK each year. Using laser, heat or microwaves, the prostate lobes are trimmed from the inside. It takes about an hour, depending on how much tissue has to be removed, and you will only be in hospital for a day or two. Revolutionary new methods use robots under computer control to guide the tool removing the prostate tissue but these are still under trial.

Rare complications

10 Some men report a period of impotence after the operation which is usually temporary and is probably psychological rather than a direct effect of surgery. Even so, for the men concerned it is a very real problem and your GP may help with expert counselling. Most effects will wear off within 2 days. In cases of complete impotence, implantable prostheses can be used. 'Retrograde ejaculation', where the sperm are directed into the bladder instead of the penis, often occurs because the one-way valve at the neck of the bladder has to be widened for the operation. It will not cause any pain or harm but it obviously can affect the number of sperm leaving the penis during ejaculation. This complication is not rare and but should not affect your enjoyment of sex. Incidentally, it is the action of this one-way valve which also prevents urine passing down the penis during ejaculation. This explains why it is difficult to pass water with a strong erection.

Prevention

11 Not knowing the cause of these conditions makes it difficult to give any solid advice on prevention, but the advice given in the next section on prostatic cancer makes good sense. Early detection is vital. With modern treatment, the outlook is often far from gloomy. Sadly, men tend to see their doctor late, making treatment difficult and less certain.

11 Cancer of the prostate

1 *Remember, cancer of the prostate can sometimes cause the same symptoms as BPH and be completely painless but early prostate cancer is almost always symptomless.* It kills around 10,000 UK men a year, which is four times the rate of female deaths from cervical cancer. It mainly affects men over the age of 65 to 70, although men as young as 55 can also develop the cancer. Survival at the age of 70 is 50 per cent. Unfortunately we do not know what causes prostate cancer, but early diagnosis is essential for successful treatment.

2 You are more at risk of developing prostate cancer if:

- A close member of your family (brother, father) has developed the cancer.
- You have high levels of testosterone.
- You are Afro-Caribbean.
- You eat a diet rich in animal products, particularly animal fat.
- You are over 70 years of age.

Prevention

3 It is interesting that men from Japan and China have the lowest rates of prostate cancer in the world and this may be a valuable clue, particularly as this protection disappears if these men move to areas with a Western diet. The role of dietary oestrogen, and traces of the same hormone picked up from pollution, is still unclear. As in many other cancers, antioxidants could be useful in preventing the disease. Vitamins E & C and beta carotene

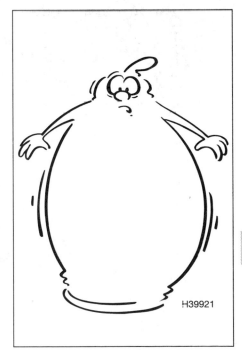

H39921

A sensible protective diet would involve weight reduction

7

mop up free radicals which damage genetic material in the cells leading to cancer. Selenium may also be a big factor, as countries with low selenium soil and thus low selenium food tend to have higher levels of prostatic cancer. Zinc is used by the body to make an enzyme which acts like a switch for certain protective genes. Red meat is considered a major factor in stimulating the cancer while nuts and seeds act as barriers. A recent report shows finesteride capable of reducing prostatic cancer by up to 25 per cent. If true, this is the single greatest ever break-though in cancer prevention by drugs. Similarly, chlamydia infection has been linked to prostate cancer in later life. Safer sex makes even more sense.

4 A sensible protective diet would involve:

- Weight reduction if you are overweight. Oestrogen levels may be elevated in obese men.
- Limit animal fat intake, and reduce all fats anyway. It should represent about 25 to 30 per cent of your energy needs.
- Eat chicken and fish instead of red meat.
- Eat at least half a kilo (one pound) of fresh fruit per day.
- Take a tip from the Orientals; eat their food.
- Eat nuts and seeds, rather than sweets.
- Increase your intake of antioxidants by eating carrots and citrus fruits.
- There is recent evidence that finesteride (used for treating BPH) may protect men from prostate cancer.

Detection

5 Along with rectal examination, your doctor can perform a blood test for enzymes released by the tumour. A recent development which identifies proteins specific to the cancer (prostate specific antigen or PSA), looks promising and may be a means of screening for the disease. Ultrasound is useful but cannot detect very early cancers of the prostate. No matter what method is used, early detection could be the key to successful treatment so if you are concerned, and particularly if you fall into the higher risk groups, you should think about seeing your doctor.

Treatment

6 Treatment can involve surgery and radiotherapy to either remove or reduce the bulk of the growth. Regular drug implants under the skin inhibit testosterone from stimulating the growth of the tumour. You will need to use these drugs for the rest of your life. Even if all of the tumour cannot be removed by surgery, this

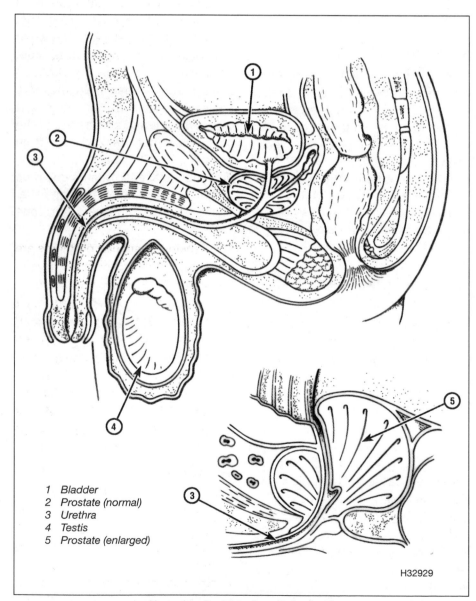

1 Bladder
2 Prostate (normal)
3 Urethra
4 Testis
5 Prostate (enlarged)

H32929

Normal and enlarged prostate gland

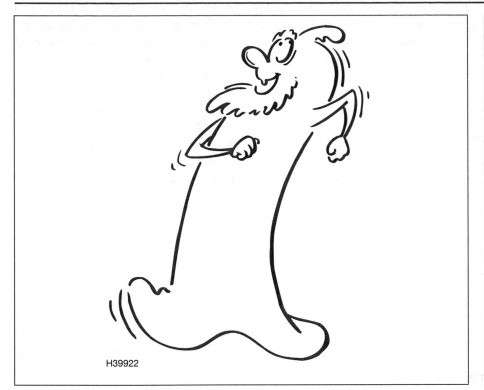

H39922

Many sufferers of prostate cancer live to a ripe old age

Dear Doctor

I understand that following a prostatectomy a man can no longer ejaculate, the semen travelling backwards into the bladder. In spite of this happening, and assuming the man's erection is as good as ever, should he still be able to enjoy a satisfying orgasm?

Prostatectomy doesn't always lead to retrograde ejaculation which you describe. In some cases the valve which controls and directs the flow of urine and sperm can be damaged during surgery. There is no change in sexual enjoyment and you can still have children through the assistance of your fertility clinic.

can slow it down quite dramatically, giving the man a relatively normal life for many years. Many sufferers live to a ripe old age, dying from something other than their prostatic cancer.

Unwanted effects of treatment

- Side effects depend upon the way the tumour is treated.
- Radiotherapy is used for early cancers or when the tumour cannot be reduced by surgery. It is also very useful in reducing pain, particularly if the tumour has settled in bone. Temporary irritation of the bladder is common, with a burning sensation when passing water. On the plus side, radiotherapy may not cause impotence.
- Surgery can damage nerves which control the erection resulting in impotence but this is less common with improved techniques.

- Hormone treatment can often result in impotence, although it is possible to implant a penile prosthesis in some cases. There are also drugs available which cause an erection when injected correctly.

Further information

7 If you would like to know more, look in the Contacts section at the back of the book, or contact:

Prostate Help Association
Langworth
Lincoln
LN3 5DF

Prostate Research Campaign UK
Canada House
272 Field End Road
Eastcote
Middlesex
HA4 9NA
020 8582 0246
www.prostate-research.org.uk
info@prostate-research.org.uk

12 Cancer of the testes

1 Thankfully testicular problems are relatively rare. Testicular cancer is the most serious. It represents only 1 per cent of all cancers in men, but it is the single biggest cause of cancer related death in men aged between 18 and 35, although it can develop in boys as young as 15. Currently about 1500 men a year develop the disease. Unfortunately the number of cases has doubled in the last 20 years and is still rising.

Symptoms

- A lump on one testicle.
- Pain and tenderness in either testicle.
- Discharge (pus or smelly goo) from the penis.
- Blood in the sperm at ejaculation.
- A build up of fluid inside the scrotum.

7

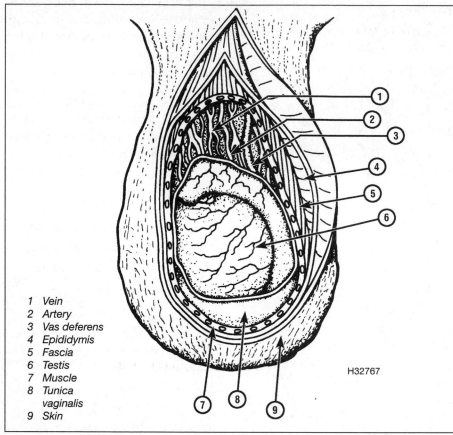

1 Vein
2 Artery
3 Vas deferens
4 Epididymis
5 Fascia
6 Testis
7 Muscle
8 Tunica
   vaginalis
9 Skin

H32767

Testis and scrotum

Dear Doctor

My normally active sex life ceased 6 months ago when I was diagnosed with haemospermia. Previously I had occasionally ejaculated blood and sperm but assumed that it was due to my partner's tight vagina and squeezing of my penis during intercourse. Hospital tests yielded nothing and no reason for my condition was given. Sometimes I have a 'wet dream' and also masturbate but any ejaculation causes discomfort for a few days. Understandably, women are put off. Can you please help.

Blood in the sperm – haemospermia – is fairly rare. It should always be investigated as it can be caused by problems with the prostate, bladder or testes. It can also be brought on by trauma. A good kick in the nether regions is a classic cause. Bicycles with crossbars will also introduce you to the condition if your feet slip out of the pedals while going up a steep hill. (That's why they are called 'cross' bars. You really are cross afterwards.) So long as nothing has been found you should still be able to enjoy sex. Condoms are essential for safer sex anyway so simply wear one when making love, even during oral sex. Blood coming into contact with your testes can lead to infertility, so you need to know where it is coming from.

- A heavy dragging feeling in the groin or scrotum.
- An increase in size of the testicle. (It is normal for one testicle to be larger then the other, but the sizes and shape should remain more or less the same.)
- An enlargement of the breasts, with or without tenderness.

Causes

2 The causes of the increase in testicular cancers are unknown. Exposure to female hormones in the environment, in water (possibly from the oral contraceptive pill contaminating water supplies), or in baby milk have been suggested. In Spain and most Asian countries there has been no significant increase but we do not know why. At the same time sperm counts are falling across Europe and this may be part of the picture. Undescended testicles are a major factor (where the testicle stays inside the body after birth and will not sit in the scrotum). Men with one or two undescended testes have a greatly increased risk – one in 44. The condition can be corrected surgically, but must be done before the age of 10.

3 Your risk increases if your father or brother suffered from testicular cancer.

Prevention

4 For once men are positively encouraged to feel themselves, but this time to do more than 'check they're still there'. Self examination is the name of the game. Check your tackle monthly like this.

5 Do it lying in a warm bath or while having a long shower, as this makes the skin of the scrotum softer and

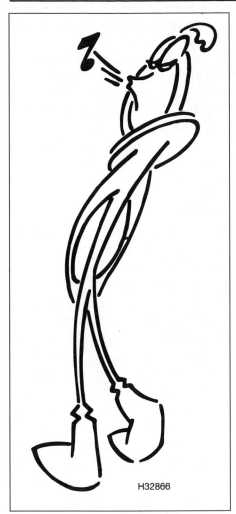

Check your tackle monthly

H32866

easier therefore, to feel the testicles inside.

6 Cradle the scrotum in the palm of your hand. Feel the difference between the testicles. You will almost definitely feel that one is larger and lying lower. This is completely normal.

7 Examine each one in turn, and then compare them with each other. Use both hands and gently roll each testicle between thumb and forefinger. Check for any lumps or swellings. Remember that the duct carrying sperm to the penis, the epididymis, normally feels bumpy. It lies along the top and back of the testis.

Dear Doctor

I have noticed a small bump on my boyfriend's testicle which seems to be getting bigger. He says it isn't painful and it is perfectly normal. I've asked him to see the doctor but he says he hasn't got time. What can I do if he won't listen to me?

If the lump is only on one side you are correct to be concerned. There are many things it can be which are fortunately not serious. On the other hand it could be something which he most definitely should get seen to. Testicular cancer is most common in young men but it is very treatable when caught early. Have a chat with your own doctor who might be able to convince him that it is in his own best interests to be examined. Ideally you should approach your boyfriend's doctor but remember, he may take exception to 'interference'. Your own doctor will give you good advice as he may know your boyfriend's GP.

Complications

8 Many types of testicular cancer can be cured in around 96 per cent of cases if caught at an early stage. Even when these tumours spread, they can still be cured in 80 per cent of cases, and large volume tumours can be cured in 60 per cent of cases. Even so, late diagnosis increases the risk of a poorer response to treatment.

9 One testicle may need to be removed, but a prosthesis (false one) disguises the fact almost completely.

10 Treatment with radiotherapy or radiography may affect your ability

to father children, but in many cases fertility is not affected. It is also possible to store sperm before treatment.

Self care

11 Too frequent self examination can actually make it more difficult to notice any difference and may cause unnecessary worry.

Dear Doctor

I'm not really sure if you can help me. My GP has refused to see me any more even though I am really worried about my testicles. He makes me very angry because I'm doing his work for him yet he won't even examine me any more when I ask him to. I check my testicles every day and I have found a number of things wrong including a lump which my GP says is just a hydrocele and is harmless. I'm still finding lumps and bumps but he ignores me. Should I complain? I'm not expecting you to stick up for me as you are a GP yourself.

Yes I am a GP as well but I can still give you objective advice. You are probably worrying far too much and examining yourself too often. As you know the surface of the testes is naturally bumpy and this is not helped if you have a hydrocele which is just a small bag of fluid in the cord which passes from the testis into the body. Complaining is not as productive as explaining to your doctor just why you are so concerned. Perhaps a brother or friend suffered from testicular cancer? Write to him first. He may refer you for a second opinion to reassure you and put your mind at ease.

7

Further information

12 If you would like to know more, look in the Contacts section at the back of the book, or contact:

The Orchid Cancer Appeal
St Bartholomew's Hospital
London, EC1A 7BE
www.orchid-cancer.org.uk
info@orchid-cancer.org.uk

TSE Testicular Self Examination Leaflets from:
Cancer Research UK
PO Box 123
Lincoln's Inn Fields
London, WC2A 3PX
020 7009 8820
www.cancerresearchuk.org

13 Vagina

1 While men invariably find fault over the size of their penis, women complain about the size of their

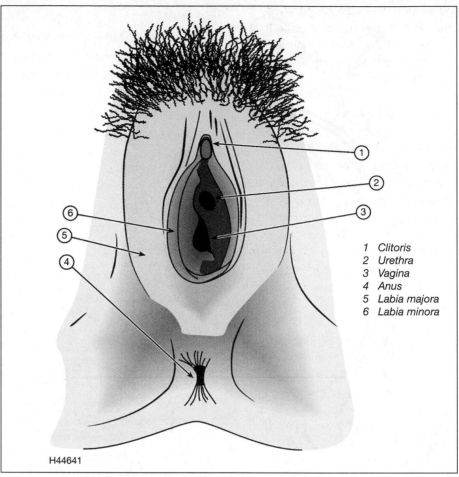

1	Clitoris
2	Urethra
3	Vagina
4	Anus
5	Labia majora
6	Labia minora

H44641

External genital features – female

Dear Doctor
I am a 27 year old woman, who happens to believe that the size of a man's penis is everything. Since the birth of my child 5 years ago I feel as though my vagina is twice as wide as before. Sex with my partner became really boring as I couldn't even feel him inside me, whereas before it was wonderful. We have split up and I have become involved with several men since, but when we have sex the size of their penis always puts me off them. I regularly do my pelvic floor exercises, but my sex life hasn't improved. I can and do enjoy sex in various ways but I think that penetration is the ultimate ingredient within a full and happy sexual relationship. Please help me. It's hard enough to find a decent man, let alone find one with all the matching vital statistics.

All over the world, men are now reading this and muttering, 'typical woman'. We are educated from puberty to believe that it's not what you've got that matters, it's what you do with it. In fact many if not most women actually do think that penis size is important. In your case you are finding fault with the whole of mankind when you have already given the explanation for your poor sexual stimulation. If the average guy in the street had to pass a rugby ball through his anus he would not be surprised if it was wider from that point on. Babies' heads are a little unforgiving on vaginas. If a tear occurred or an episiotomy was performed, the tightness of your vagina will depend to some extent on how well they were repaired by stitching. Pelvic floor exercises will help, but if the increase in size is considerable you need to practise different positions. The 'cat' position, where the man lies higher up while face to face, helps press the penis against the clitoris. If all else fails you would probably be better seeking advice from a plastic surgeon or obstetrician than wearing out and demoralising half the male population.

vaginas *and* the size of penises. It is not PC these days to say that the size of a man's penis is everything, but to some women it most definitely is.

2 People can be so hurtful, often without any realisation of the pain they have just caused with a throwaway remark. Women are every bit as conscious about their vaginas as men during their development. Nature can also be cruel and different rates of growth, along with the natural variation in sizes, can make a young woman's imagination and confidence go into a downward spiral.

3 The vagina is essentially a blind ending tube. With vigorous love making air is forced in which causes it to balloon somewhat. This is more common if the muscles which surround the vagina are lax, say after childbirth. Pelvic floor exercises to strengthen the pubocoxygeal muscles can help.

Dear Doctor

Whenever my boyfriend and I have sex, my vagina becomes loose after a couple of minutes. This makes it difficult for both of us to achieve orgasm as it feels like there is no contact. Is there anything I can do to prevent this happening? Please help as it's ruining our sex life.

Imagine you are about to pass water. Bear down while at the same time use your pelvic muscles to stop yourself actually wetting yourself. You can do these exercises anywhere, any time, but you do tend to attract unwanted attention while at the bus stop.

Dear Doctor

I have a really stringy piece of skin on my vaginal lip. I have one child and sometimes try and blame it on having a baby as they stitched me up after I gave birth. But I also think it had something to do with the way my ex-partner liked to really push his penis inside me. Please help and tell me what you know about the problem I have.

Most of us are actually unaware how our vital bits look and what is normal. The vagina has a number of labia which can be mistaken for abnormal 'flaps'. As vaginas were designed for penises it is unlikely that your partner caused this flap through intercourse, unless he was extremely violent. It may also be the result of childbirth although such irregularities generally resolve themselves with time. Episiotomy repairs were once carried out by junior staff. They considered it part of their practice in learning how to stitch wounds. Times change and now only senior staff or those under direct supervision perform this most delicate task. It is possible that the flap on your vagina may have resulted from poor technique. It is also possible that it came from tearing of the vagina during childbirth. Either way it can be corrected by simple surgery. Ask your GP for an appointment with the consultant who was in charge of your pregnancy and delivery.

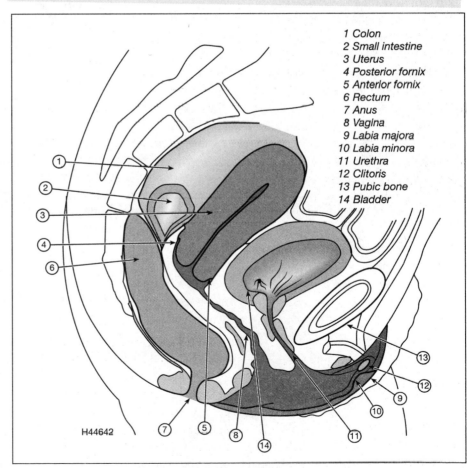

1 Colon
2 Small intestine
3 Uterus
4 Posterior fornix
5 Anterior fornix
6 Rectum
7 Anus
8 Vagina
9 Labia majora
10 Labia minora
11 Urethra
12 Clitoris
13 Pubic bone
14 Bladder

H44642

Lower female abdomen

7

4 There are some beautiful stories going around about men and women who become locked in place during intercourse. Most of these come from the same stable as the ones about women having teeth in their vagina. Even so, spasm of the vaginal muscles can cause problems, as can the terminology.

> Dear Doctor
>
> I am a 21 year old woman who is very confused. I have got a couple of really embarrassing things wrong with me which might not be as serious as I think. When I have sex with my partner I suffer a lot of pain. A doctor told me I have vaginismus. What exactly is this?

Vaginismus is common. It is not caused by any physical disorder. Anxiety, dryness or lack of foreplay can result in a spasm of the muscles which surrounds the vagina. Stories about men being trapped in women's vaginas because of this spasm make great reading in the tabloids but have little basis in truth. What vaginismus does cause is pain on intercourse which can create a vicious circle of anxiety, dryness then muscle spasm. Each time it happens it serves only to reinforce the expectation that it will always happen. Forget about penetrative sex for a while. Use mutual masturbation and other forms of sexual play instead. Once penetrative sex comes back on the scene use plenty of foreplay and lubrication.

5 Have you ever watched a romantic film where two lovers are lying on the beach? At just the right moment great crashing waves substitute for what the film censors saw but thought was unfit for everyone else. What we also don't see are two people walking like John Wayne afterwards as sand can get in the most sensitive places. Load bearing surfaces become worn and rough, ask any mechanic. Nature has its own way of ensuring a smooth ride, as it were. Unfortunately there are plenty of things which will throw sand into the works. On the other hand, there also plenty of ways of getting it out again.

> Dear Doctor
>
> Please could you help me. I am 47 and have a very dry vagina and I now don't get aroused when I have sex with my husband. We used to be able to do it any time and anywhere. I have been put on HRT as the doctor thinks I've started the menopause.

Your doctor may have performed a blood test to find out if you are going through the menopause. There is a significant drop in oestrogen levels when the menopause starts. Vaginal dryness is common during this phase as the lining is maintained to some extent by oestrogen stimulation. Hormone replacement therapy may relieve this. If one form of treatment fails you should consider others before abandoning HRT completely as there are different combinations of hormones. Meantime, break the vicious circle by trying more non-penetrative sex, longer foreplay and using lubricating creams.

6 Sex is noisy. Doing it quietly is something younger people try to master but usually fail, especially when their parents are within earshot. Parents are generally more adept at it, knowing that the slightest indication of being awake will lead to a passion-crushing avalanche of children wanting milk-shakes for breakfast.

> Dear Doctor
>
> I am just screaming with embarrassment, but I don't know where to turn. My new man and I are about to make love for the first time but I am so scared about it, because – to put it bluntly – I break wind all the time during sex. From the front! I know what you'll say, just laugh it all off and it will be fine but you don't understand. It happens so often. I wrap my legs around my boyfriend's neck as he prepares to enter me and . . . then it happens. I think I will die of shame. Please, please, please help me.

I once knew a student who could do passable rendition of the Blaydon Races in just the same way. It was a party piece which made her very popular. I never actually took her home to meet mum and dad as they were both tone deaf. Air trapped in the vagina only has one way out. During intercourse air is pushed in, only to be released just when you could do without the noise. I am informed that non-circumcised men tend to cause this more often, as the foreskin acts like a piston ring. Sex is noisy. A sense of humour is essential for love play. You are anxiously waiting for it to occur which makes you tense and more likely to retain air. Light-heartedly mention it to your boyfriend and if he is any kind of decent guy he will laugh.

14 Pubic hair

1 Hair is funny stuff. We are constantly bemoaning its loss, change in colour or being found in the 'wrong' position. Despite being perfectly natural, dark hair on a woman's upper lip is considered unsightly in some cultures. On the other hand, lack of hair either on the head or around the vagina is considered equally unacceptable in others. Prostitutes in the middle ages used pubic wigs to mask any visible signs of sexually transmitted disease such as syphilis. This went to the opposite in the 1980s of shaving the pubic hair into extinction. It is impossible to satisfy all the different perceptions of what is beautiful or normal. Thankfully what turns one person right off is a green light for sex to others. There is a hairy place for all of us.

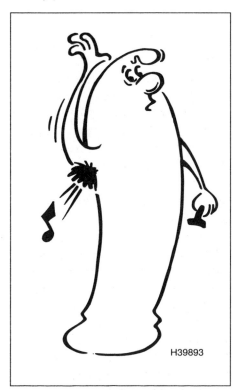

H39893

Some people like wind whistling through the hairy bits

Dear Doctor

I have just started seeing a new woman, we've been getting on really well and I thought everything was going well. Our sexual chemistry was really running high and neither of us could wait until we first had sex. But when it came to the crunch and we were undressing, I found out that she had shaved her pubic hair. I thought she was a really nice girl and I really fancy her a lot but surely this is a bit weird? I don't really go for it at all as I think it's a bit strange. I do want to try and understand because I like her a lot, but I couldn't ask her in case she gets offended. What should I do?

Many women shave their pubic hair, or at least the bits which show around a bikini bottom. Some women think shaving their pubic hair makes them appear younger, and sexier. Simply telling your girlfriend that you prefer her au naturel will save her all that work in the bath. She may be relieved to hear it.

15 Clitoris

1 The foetus decides which sex it is going to be rather late in development and so both sets of reproductive organs develop. Once it has made up its mind which colour booties it will be wearing once born, the foetus suppresses the set of organs belonging to the opposite sex. They still remain, if only in a rudimentary form. The clitoris is therefore the remains of what would in a male foetus have developed into a penis.

2 It is possible for a person to have both sets of sexual organs. Although this is seen more often nowadays, it is still rare.

Dear Doctor

The problem is that I think my clitoris is too big, as my school friend showed me hers and I could hardly see it. Normally mine is about an inch long but when I get aroused it becomes quite hard and sticks out. My boyfriend thinks I am deformed and says that I have a penis. Am I deformed? Will I have to have an operation?

The clitoris is anatomically the equivalent of the male penis, so your boyfriend is correct. All women have a penis, just as all men have nipples. The clitoris is an erectile organ so should get bigger on arousal. Like other sex organs it only really fully develops at puberty, so your friend may not yet have her full complement of sex hormones in circulation. There is no 'normal' size for a clitoris and large ones are considered highly attractive to most men. If you really cannot stand its appearance plastic surgery might help but would be expensive and most surgeons would be reluctant to perform the operation, particularly on a young woman. You boyfriend needs to be your ex-boyfriend as soon as possible, but before he goes, you should just whisper in his ear that his penis reminds you of an average-sized clitoris.

7

Chapter 8
Sexually Transmitted Infections

Contents

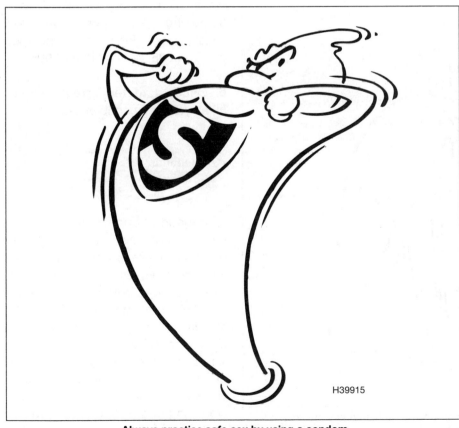

Always practise safe sex by using a condom

1 Introduction

1 Sexually transmitted infections (STIs) can affect you at any age, whether you're straight or gay, in a long-term relationship or with a casual partner. Symptoms don't always show up immediately, so you could have been infected recently or a long time ago. It is important to ensure that you always practise safer sex by using a condom, unless and until you are in a steady relationship with one partner, neither of you having sex with anyone else and sure that neither of you is infected. (So, always use a condom, yes?)

2 If you haven't practised safer sex in the past and are worried that you may have caught an STI, you can have a confidential check-up and treatment if needed.

8

Your choice for treatment

3 You can attend either your own doctor or the local genitourinary medicine (GUM) or STI clinic, which will be located at one of the major hospitals in your area. Confidentiality is all-important at these clinics. Call NHS Direct for details of your nearest clinic. You will need to be honest about your symptoms to the doctor who asks you questions, as it can be impossible to work out what is wrong without the correct information. You can remain anonymous if you feel more comfortable, although there is no chance of the fact of your attendance going any further, even to your GP, let alone any diagnosis that may be made.

4 Certain tests may be needed to make an accurate diagnosis, although it may be fairly obvious on your first visit and the treatment may start immediately with no return needed. It is worth remembering that the doctors and nurses who staff these clinics are professionals who see you simply as a person who, like a patient with any other illness, needs treatment.

2 Chlamydia

1 Non-specific urethritis, which simply means an inflammation or infection of the urethra, is an all-embracing term which includes infection by chlamydia. Men and women suffering from this infection may complain of an intense burning sensation when passing water. There may also be a white discharge. The condition is often free of symptoms in women and in men.

2 Chlamydia actually causes few problems for men other than this discomfort, but can be disastrous if it is passed on to women. It is the single biggest cause of infection of the fallopian tubes (pelvic inflammatory disease), leading to infertility and ectopic pregnancy (a potentially lethal condition where the baby attaches to the wall of the fallopian tube instead of the wall of the womb). It can also cause blindness and pneumonia in a child born to an infected woman.

3 Condoms provide almost total protection.

Detection and treatment

4 Chlamydia is detected by taking a urine sample. The Department of Health is planning to introduce a screening programme, targeted initially at females between the ages of 16 and 25, during 2004 / 2005.

5 Once detected, treatment of chlamydia is by antibiotics.

3 Hepatitis

1 Although hepatitis is one of the more deadly sexually transmitted diseases, there is now a protective vaccine to prevent some forms of it. Even so, the number of infected people is rising steadily and currently stands at roughly 700 men each year. It can cause as little as a flu-like illness or as much as total destruction of the liver. Typically, it will cause varying degrees of jaundice (yellowing of the skin and the whites of the eyes). This is caused by the

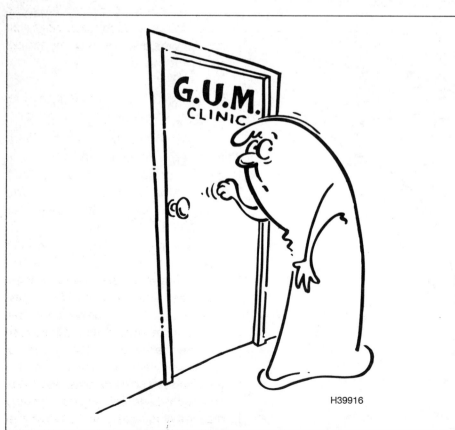

H39916

You can attend either your own doctor or the local genitourinary medical clinic (GUM)

build-up of a pigment which is normally broken down by the liver.

2 Hepatitis is transmitted in the same way as HIV, i.e. via bodily fluids. It only requires a tiny fraction of a drop of blood to transmit the disease. For this reason it can be caught from sharing a toothbrush or kissing when there is bleeding from the gums. Worse still, the virus can survive a week or more in the dried state and so can be picked up from, for instance, a razor.

3 There is no way of knowing if the person with whom you are having sex harbours the infection. The incubation period, i.e., how long it takes before the illness manifests itself, is six months from infection. Some people can 'carry' the virus and yet not exhibit the condition.

4 Most people will not require immunisation, but depending upon your lifestyle it may be wise to consult your GP.

4 Genital herpes

1 This is the third most common STI. It is caused by the Herpes Simplex Virus (HSV).

2 The virus comes in two forms, HSV I and HSV II. Both are likely to infect parts of the body where two types of skin meet together - typically the corners of the mouth, the outer parts of the genital areas and even the anus. Both cause crusted blisters and then ulcers that weep a thin, watery substance. This substance is highly infectious, since it contains the virus that causes the condition. The attacks can last for months and then disappear for years, or even never return. Stress and coincidental illness can also bring on attacks.

3 You are definitely infectious during the presence of the sores.

Even when sores are not present, it might be possible to pass on the infection. For some people, the condition will pass unnoticed, with only tiny ulcers on the penis to show its presence.

4 You need to avoid all sexual activity if you are having an attack, as this means you are highly infectious. At other times the use of condoms gives maximum protection for your partner. Condoms with a spermicide appear to offer greater protection than those without.

Treatment

5 Anti-viral drugs can be applied directly to the affected skin or taken orally. They are most effective if used before the sores break out. This is signalled by a tingling, itchy, painful sensation in the affected area. They are only effective during the first attack in some people and have not been shown to have any impact on subsequent attacks.

6 Roughly 50% of people who have had one attack never have another. Unfortunately, it is impossible to completely get rid of the virus.

5 Genital warts

1 Papilloma viruses, which cause warts, can affect any part of the skin. The virus can be transmitted by physical contact including sexual intercourse. Like the warts commonly seen on people's hands, genital warts can vary in size from tiny skin tags to large fungating masses like cauliflowers. While the latter are hard to miss, the less obvious form can be prevented from

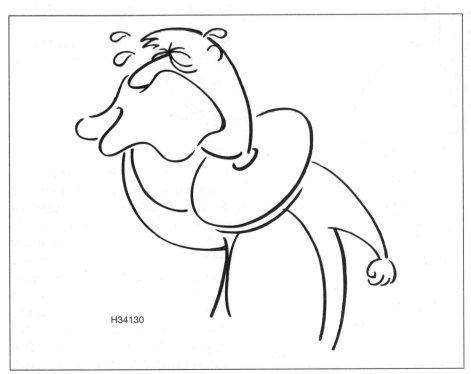

H34130

Hepatitis can cause anything from a flu-like illness to destruction of the liver

8

causing infection only by covering the area completely.

2 One in eight people attending GUM clinics have genital warts. Around 100,000 people are treated for these warts each year in the UK; many more may simply put up with them, and many people do not even know they have them.

3 Genital warts may be a factor in causing cervical cancer in women and rectal cancer in both sexes.

Treatment

4 There are drugs which can be applied directly to warts which will cause them to disappear. Liquid nitrogen is now used less often as it can leave a painful 'burn' in such sensitive areas. Genital warts usually cause little discomfort, although they are often itchy and may bleed with scratching. Use a condom to prevent catching them in the first place.

6 Syphilis

1 A potentially serious condition, syphilis was almost extinct but is now on the increase in the UK. It is caused by a spirochete, a microscopic parasite which is highly infectious. Many people are unaware of the infection, but if it is not treated it can develop over a number of years into a condition which can affect the heart and brain. It can also be passed from a pregnant woman to her child.

2 The first sign of infection is an ulcer called a chancre which appears on the penis, the mouth, or in or around the vagina. The ulcer is usually painless so it may pass unnoticed. The second stage of infection produces a characteristic skin rash. Sufferers are infectious during both these stages.

3 The parasite cannot pass through a condom, so this will give almost 100% protection.

Treatment

4 Penicillin is given as a single large dose by injection to any part of the body and will almost invariably cure the condition if it is caught in the early stages.

7 Trichomoniasis

1 This microscopic parasite lives in the urinary tract. It can cause pain when passing water, but can also be completely symptomless. When it has no effect on the male partner but the female partner complains of a smelly green discharge from the vagina, tests may show its presence in the man.

2 Condoms prevent the transmission of the parasite.

Treatment

3 The parasite is sensitive to antibiotics.

8 Gonorrhoea

1 Caused by a bacterium, this disease is sometimes misdiagnosed as it can often give only minimum symptoms. It is commonly known as the clap, possibly from the French words *clapoir* meaning sexual sore,

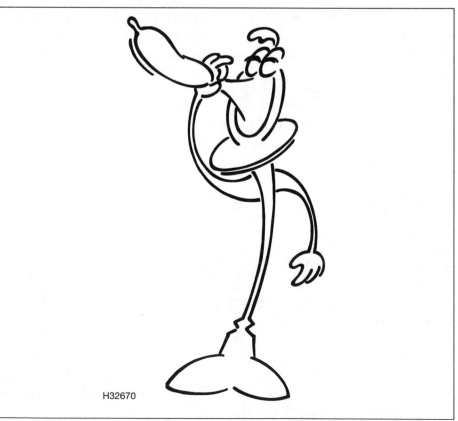

H32670

If you're going to have a bang, make sure you have airbag protection

or *clapier*, old-fashioned slang for a brothel.

2 Gonorrhoea is not rare. It can cause a yellow/white discharge from the penis or vagina, along with pain on passing water. When infecting the anus there can be a similar discharge. Most of the symptoms of infection will start within 5 days of infection and include a vague ache of the joints and muscles. Although these can disappear after a further 10 or so days, the person remains infectious. It can cause reduced fertility if not treated.

3 As usual, condoms provide almost 100% protection.

Treatment

2 Antibiotics are effective, although the emergence of antibiotic-resistant strains of the bacterium may mean that more than one antibiotic has to be tried.

9 HIV & AIDS

1 Infection with the human immunodeficiency virus (HIV) reduces the number of white blood cells, thus lowering the body's resistance to infection. At the time of writing at least 13 million people in the world were HIV positive. Although the virus only appeared in the UK in 1982 there are over 4,000 new cases reported each year, with perhaps 10 times this number unrecognised. But it is not all doom and gloom. New treatments are significantly extending life expectancy. Even so, the name of the game is prevention.

Symptoms

2 Early stages of infection generally go unnoticed and it needs an antibody test from a blood or saliva sample to confirm the presence of the virus. The appearance of the antibodies can take months and is known as seroconversion. A vague non-specific illness similar to flu or glandular fever sometimes follows the infection at around 6 to 7 weeks later. A variable period of time, years even, can then pass completely symptom free. The occurrence of oral thrush, persistent herpes (cold sores), or strange chest infections which clear only slowly with treatment, are ominous signs of the body's declining ability to fight off other infections.

Causes

3 Body fluids are often cited as the carrier of the virus. Actually this can be narrowed down to blood, semen and saliva. Although the risk of infection from saliva is extremely small it makes sense to avoid obvious risks such as oral sex without adequate protection. Similarly, there are no cases of doctors passing on the virus to their patient, although a number of doctors have suffered from infection in the opposite direction. The main routes of infection are:

- Sexual transmission via blood from small cuts either in the mouth (oral sex), vagina, anus or penis. Sexual orientation is not exclusive, with both gay and straight men at risk.
- Blood transfusion in countries with poor medical resources is still a risk; you can buy a travel kit from your GP.
- Sharing dirty needles or even razor blades.

Prevention

4 According to the World Health Organisation (WHO) up to 90 per cent of those people infected in the world have contracted HIV through heterosexual sex of whatever form. Dental dams and male and female condoms, particularly those containing the spermicide non-oxynol-9, give a high degree of protection.

5 If extra lubrication is required, do not use oil-based lubricants such as Vaseline, baby oil, margarine or butter. They will damage the condom. There are water-based lubricants available. If you are not sure, ask the chemist, they sell thousands of them and will not be embarrassed to give advice.

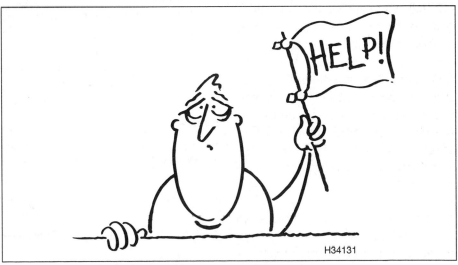

H34131

If you're unsure which condom or lubricant to use, ask the pharmacist

8

Self care

6 Healthy diets are not quite the same when you are HIV positive. Cutting back on your fat intake will reduce your chances of having an early heart attack at, say, 60 years. Common-sense will indicate how useful such a diet will be to an HIV infected person, depending upon their age at infection. In fact, full fat milk, cheeses, creamy yoghurt, butter and ice-cream are all preferable to their low fat alternatives. Fat supplies not only a valuable energy source but also vitamins which are only found in fatty products.

Further information

7 If you would like to know more, look in the Contacts section at the back of the book, or contact:

Black HIV-AIDS Network Limited
St Stephens House
41 Uxbridge Road
London
W12 8LH
Tel 020 8749 2828

Body Positive
51b Philbeach Gardens
Earls Court
London
SW5 9EB
Tel 020 7835 1045

The National AIDS Helpline
Tel 0800 567 123 (English, Chinese, Cantonese)
Tel 0800 282 445 (English, Bengali, Hindu, Punjabi and Urdu)
www.playingsafely.co.uk

Terrence Higgins Trust
Monday-Friday 10am-10pm,
Saturday-Sunday Noon-6pm
Tel 0171 242 1010
www.tht.org.uk

10 Thrush

1 *Candida albicans* is a fungus which is normally present on or in various parts of the body, including the skin, digestive tract and vagina, without causing any problems. For various reasons it can sometimes grow rapidly and cause thrush. Both men and women can suffer from thrush, but it is more common in women.

Symptoms in women

- A creamy thick white vaginal discharge.
- Itchiness and irritation of the vagina.
- Pain or burning after passing water.

Symptoms in men

- Itchiness and irritation of the tip of the penis, or under the foreskin.
- Red patches on the tip of the penis.
- A thick, creamy discharge under the foreskin, which may also be difficult to retract.

Causes

- A prolonged course of antibiotics.
- The oral contraceptive pill.
- Hormonal changes preceding the period.
- Steroid treatment.
- Diabetes.
- Immune system problems.
- Sex with an infected person.

Prevention

- After being on the toilet, women should always wipe from front to back.
- Change underwear frequently, particularly after exercise.
- Choose cotton rather than nylon pants.
- Avoid harsh soaps, they kill the good bacteria which prevent thrush.

Complications

- Thankfully there are few serious complications of thrush. It can, however, make life very miserable. Sex can be painful, likewise passing water.

Self care

- Eat live ('bio') yoghurt and apply it to the affected area. It will replace the missing Lactobacillus which prevents thrush.
- Ask your pharmacist for anti-fungal preparations.
- Your partner may need treatment as well.

See your doctor

- If thrush keeps coming back for no apparent reason.
- If the discharge changes in smell or appearance.
- If there is any abdominal pain.

Chapter 9
Conception and contraception

Contents

1 Timing is everything

Introduction

1 Choosing the time of being a dad may not always be in your control, but if it is, there are advantages and disadvantages for young dad versus old dad.

Teenage dad

2 Becoming a parent in your teens is generally best avoided if possible. Research shows that teenage mothers are significantly disadvantaged with regard to their standard of living later in life; teenage dads probably aren't much better off.

Young dad

3 You are going to need all the youth you can muster, especially in the first few weeks when the jet lag from the lack of sleep starts to kick in. On the other hand you will be able to take part in their games as they get older without snapping your Achilles tendon and be young enough to enjoy regained independence once they leave home. You are also less likely to employ a crowbar to lever the remaining son out of the family home. Before you shout 'brace yourself darling' just a word in your ear. You may be losing the best years of your life. Along comes responsibility, a whole new look at car maintenance for necessity not fun, lost mates, especially the car maintenance variety, financial commitments when your earning power is at its lowest and of course that haunting fragrance of damp nappy.

Middle-aged dad

4 It's easy to see the advantages of kids while you are in your thirties with more earning power, a good taste of the free unfettered youth, and your parents still around to do all the baby sitting while you swan off to breakaway holidays in the Antipodes but wait a second, mate. Work pressure is at its highest during your middle age especially with jobs under pressure from women. The life long post is no more. Keeping on track with your career might be difficult with a few kids in the equation. Paradoxically you might spend more time securing their future than actually being with them.

Older dad

5 We value age as a source of wisdom and patience and of course it is theoretically possible to become a dad no matter how old you are. You don't even need to worry about the sweaty bit either, even if masturbation is not possible through erectile dysfunction. Prostatic

9

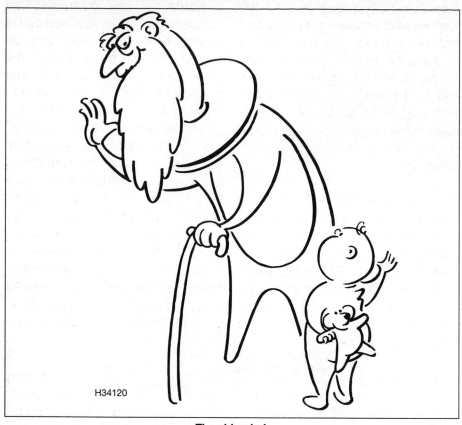

H34120

The older dad

and lessening the burden of responsibility.

6 Just a thought however before dispensing with the Zimmer for a few vital moments. Death, the grim reaper, is more likely to rob your children of your presence at an earlier age. You are less likely to take part in their activities and conception may be more difficult. There is also an increased risk of genetic malformation. Even so, average life expectancy is increasing and the older dad of the industrial revolution with a life expectancy of less than 40 years, is the middle-aged father of today.

7 Perhaps not having too much control over the matter is better in the end.

2 Getting started

Introduction

1 Ovulation usually occurs somewhere between 12 and 16 days

massage can often produce sufficient ejaculate for assisted insemination. Finance is also usually less of a problem and your decision to have kids is less likely to be based on an irrational red haze. Smaller family size is also more likely, increasing personal contact

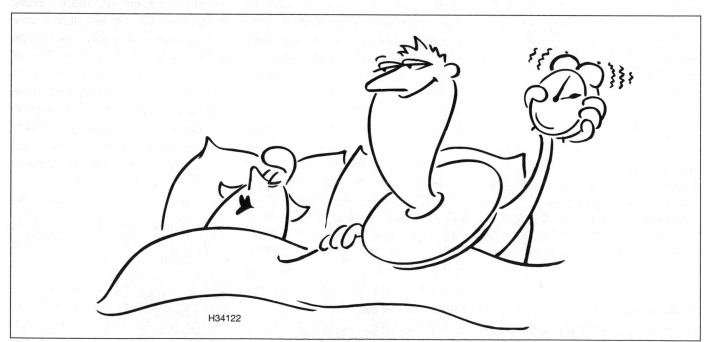

H34122

Ovulation time

before the start of the next menstrual period. This is known as the fertile period and it is during this time that the egg can be fertilised. If your partner has regular periods, this point can be worked out with reasonable accuracy by calculating backwards from when the next period is expected. Ovulation can be detected by a change in body temperature but this indicator is usually used when trying to avoid a pregnancy as it tells you that ovulation has already occurred. A change in the degree of stickiness of the mucus on the cervix is a better indicator that ovulation is about to take place. There are self-test ovulation kits available from your pharmacist that determine when ovulation is likely to happen. These are expensive and there is little evidence that they actually increase the chance of becoming pregnant any sooner then it would happen normally. Luckily, pinpointing the exact fertile period is not necessary for most people as sperm have the ability to stay alive inside the woman for several days. Therefore sex 2-3 times a week throughout the cycle will maximise the chance of achieving a pregnancy by ensuring that sperm are ready and waiting for when the egg is released.

Self help

2 There are some things you and your partner can do to help you be fit and healthy for pregnancy. Rubella infection in pregnancy can harm a developing baby, so your partner should check with her doctor to see if she needs a vaccination before you try for a pregnancy.

3 Women planning a baby should take 400 micrograms (0.4 mg) of folic acid every day from the time they stop using contraception until the 12th week of pregnancy, as folic acid reduces the risk of a baby having neural tube defects, such as spina bifida. (Those who have previously had a child with spina bifida or those who are taking drugs for epilepsy need to take bigger doses. Ask your doctor.) You can get folic acid from pharmacies.

4 A balanced diet with as much fresh food as possible will ensure enough vitamins and minerals are eaten. Soft cheeses, pâtés, soft-boiled eggs, cold prepared meats and cook-chilled foods should be avoided as there is a small risk of them being contaminated with listeria which can cause birth defects. Too much Vitamin A can be harmful to a developing baby, so pregnant women are advised not to eat liver or take Vitamin A tablets.

5 Both you and your partner should try to give up smoking, as smoking is known to carry risks for the developing baby and also to newborn babies. This is just as important for men, as smokers tend to produce fewer sperm and have more damaged sperm. Quitline can give you both help and advice on how to give up smoking.

6 Heavy or frequent drinking can harm the baby's development. Alcohol should therefore be limited to no more than one or two units of alcohol once or twice a week. If you need advice on drinking phone NHS Direct or Drinkline.

7 Weight can affect fertility by interfering with ovulation. Women who are very underweight or overweight might want to talk to NHS Direct or their practice nurse.

8 Some sexually-transmitted infections (eg, chlamydia) can cause fertility problems, some can be passed to the baby during the pregnancy or at birth (eg, HIV) and some are thought to be linked with miscarriage or premature birth (eg, trichomonas and syphilis). Many of the infections have no symptoms so if you or your partner are worried that you may have caught a sexually-transmitted infection either recently or in the past, go to a genito-urinary medicine (GUM) clinic or sexual health clinic. The service is completely free and confidential. Most large hospitals have a GUM clinic – phone Sexual Health Direct or NHS Direct for details of your nearest clinic.

9 Women should avoid changing cat litter, wear gloves when gardening, and wash hands thoroughly after handling cooked meat. This prevents infection with a parasite (toxoplasmosis) which can harm a developing baby. It Is also best to avoid X-rays and taking medication when you are pregnant or trying for a baby. Ask your doctor or a pharmacist if you need to do either of these.

10 Reducing the number of times you have sex to 'build up' a reservoir of sperm is not necessary. Sperm are produced constantly and each ejaculation contains many millions of sperm – more than enough to fertilise an egg. It is also not necessary to have sex every day, 2-3 times a week is plenty to achieve a pregnancy.

11 Not all couples achieve a pregnancy straight away so don't panic if it doesn't happen quickly as most couples get there within a year

9

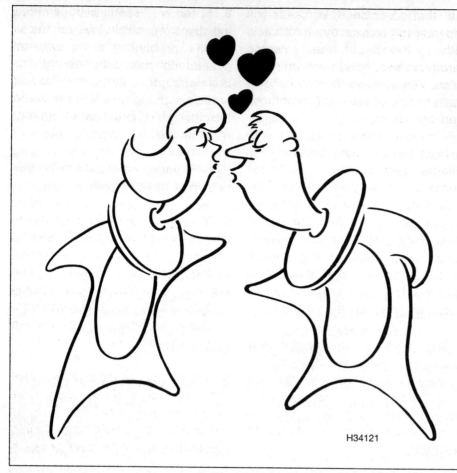

Getting started

H34121

Dear Doctor

I am single at the moment but want to be a father eventually. The problem is that I cannot ejaculate more than three times and I fear this puts the chance of pregnancy at risk. I am epileptic and my GP has said that I could be put on a pill to help with the sexual problem. However, in order for that to be done the anti-convulsive drugs I'm on would have to be changed and as my fits have been well balanced for a long time, I don't want to risk upsetting that. Is there any other way to deal with this problem.

A great deal depends upon what you mean by only being able to ejaculate three times. If this is every night you are a lucky man, but this will restrict rather than enhance your chances of fatherhood. Sperm are produced at a more or less constant rate. By ejaculating more often you deplete your store of sperm. It is better to go for more, less often. Sperm counts are dropping all over Europe and we don't know why. Artificial oestrogens in plastics and drinking water pollution may be the cause. Epilepsy in men or women is not a bar to children. Talk to your GP.

or so. Best just to try and be relaxed and enjoy not having worry about contraception for a while.

Results

12 Testing for pregnancy is simple and accurate (see Section 4).

13 All pregnancies are followed by careful monitoring through regular visits to the doctor or midwife, ultrasound and a range of other tests where necessary, so the chances of serious problems with the birth or the baby are low.

Further information

14 If you would like to know more, look in the Contacts section at the back of the book, or contact:

NHS Direct
Tel 0845 46 47
www.nhsdirect.nhs.uk

**Sexual Health Direct
(Run by the Family Planning Association)**
Tel 0845 310 1334
Mon-Fri 9am-7pm
www.fpa.org.uk

Alcoholics anonymous
Tel 01904 644026
www.alcoholics-anonymous.org

Drinkline
Tel 0800 917 8282
www.downyourdrink.org/drinkline.html
www.wrecked.co.uk

Quitline
Tel 0800 00 22 00
12am-9pm
www.quit.org.uk

Epilepsy Action
0808 800 5050
www.epilepsy.org.uk

3 How to get there

Technical specs for pregnancy

1 Technically, and by definition, pregnancy starts at the moment a sperm penetrates an egg. For practical reasons the start of pregnancy is taken from the first day of the last menstrual period, rather than from the date of fertilization. Labour and the delivery of the baby can be expected 280 days (40 weeks) from the start of the last period. The length of pregnancy may, however, vary between about 37 and 42 weeks. This variation is the cause of more fear, angst and superstition than just about anything else to do with pregnancy.

2 Sperm can carry either an X chromosome or a Y chromosome. If an X fertilizes, the result will be a girl; if Y the result will be a boy. Sperm and eggs each contain 23 chromosomes. This is half the full number. So when a sperm and an egg fuse, the full complement of chromosomes is made up, and fertilization is said to have occurred, giving the normal 46 chromosomes. Some genetic defects are linked to extra or missing chromosomes.

3 In a normal body cell, there are 46 chromosomes containing all the genetic information and arranged in 23 pairs. One set of 23 comes from the father, the other set from the mother. A fertilized ovum (egg) with its 23 pairs of chromosomes, starts to divide, rapidly and repeatedly. Every time a cell divides and reproduces, the 46 chromosomes are copied precisely.

4 Humans generally produce one baby at a time but sometimes after the first division the cells will separate to produce two individuals with exactly the same chromosomes. These are identical twins. Very rarely, this may happen again to one of the eggs, producing identical triplets.

5 Fertilization usually occurs in the fallopian tube which connects the womb to the ovary and the resulting embryo passes into the womb and begins to implant into the womb inner lining. At once the embryo sends out tiny finger-like processes called chorionic villi which help to anchor it into the womb lining and which later become the placenta.

6 Very soon, usually within one week, these villi are producing a hormone called human chorionic gonadotrophin. This prevents the body from going through menstruation which would end the pregnancy.

7 At ten weeks, the baby is about the size of your little toe and has all the recognizable external characteristics of a human male or female. At this stage the face is formed but the eyelids are fused together. The brain is in a very primitive state.

8 After three months, the baby is as long as your little finger.

9 In the sixth month, the baby is longer than your middle finger and weighs up to 800 g. Survival outside of the womb is very unlikely. The chances of survival increase rapidly with increasing maturity and most babies over 1000 g (1 kg) now do well in an intensive care ward.

10 The womb (uterus) steadily grows with the baby and eventually rises inside the abdomen. The baby is surrounded by a fluid-filled double membrane, the inner layer of which

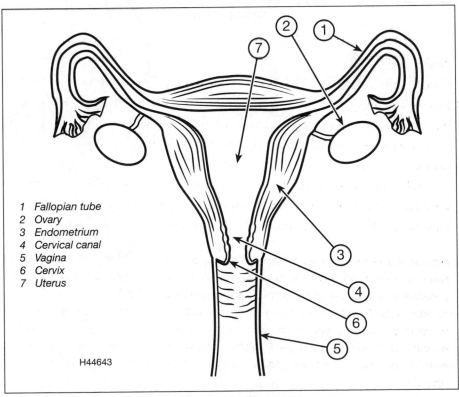

1 Fallopian tube
2 Ovary
3 Endometrium
4 Cervical canal
5 Vagina
6 Cervix
7 Uterus

H44643

Female reproductive organs

9

is called the amnion. The membrane normally ruptures and releases the amniotic fluid ('breaking of the waters') before the baby is born.

11 Around one litre of amniotic fluid fills the womb in which the baby floats freely. This fluid is protective and is constantly swallowed and then excreted as urine by the baby, so it contains material from which much information about the health of the baby can be obtained. Samples can be obtained through a needle in the procedure called amniocentesis.

12 The placenta is a thick, disc-shaped object about the size of your hand. The mother's blood enters the placenta from the womb side and the umbilical cord comes off from the free surface. In the placenta, the maternal blood comes into close contact with, but does not mix with, the foetal blood, which is being pumped through the placenta by the foetal heart.

13 A large number of nutrients and gases such as oxygen, carbon dioxide, sugars, amino acids, fats, vitamins, minerals, as well as many drugs, pass freely across the placental barrier. It is in this way that the baby is provided with all necessary supplies for maintenance as well as for body growth, and is able to get rid of waste substances.

4 Confirmation of pregnancy

1 Testing for pregnancy used to involve rabbits. Things have progressed and now the tests depend on the presence of human chorionic gonadotrophin (see *How to get there*). This hormone is produced by the developing embryo and is first present in the blood, but soon afterwards appears in the urine. A simple dipstick test into fresh urine can detect pregnancy with about a 98 per cent certainty from the time of the first missed period. There are even more sensitive immunological tests which can confirm pregnancy within a week of conception. These are normally done in a hospital laboratory and are usually used when a woman has had fertility treatment. If these tests are positive the accuracy is nearly 100 per cent certain; if the test is negative, about 80 per cent certain.

2 Pregnancy testing kits are available over-the-counter from pharmacies. (Some pharmacies will do the test for you, which can be cheaper than buying a whole testing kit.) The important thing about home testing kits is that the instructions are followed carefully otherwise you can get a wrong result. Free pregnancy testing is also available at most GPs, family planning clinics and NHS Walk-in centres.

3 A missed period is a common sign of pregnancy (however it is not the only reason women miss periods). Other signs and symptoms of pregnancy are tiredness, hunger, nausea and vomiting, frequently passing urine, changes in the breasts and low abdominal pain like a period pain. Many women can tell they are pregnant even before they have had a test performed or have missed a period.

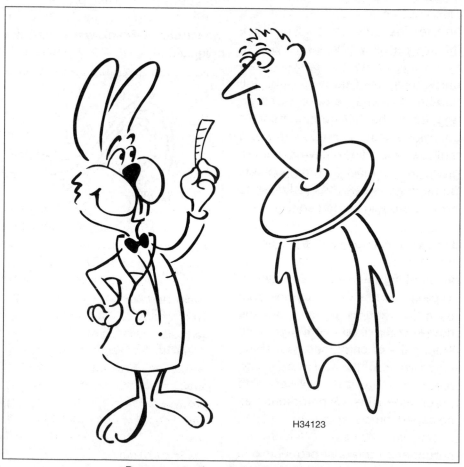

H34123

Pregnancy testing used to involve rabbits

5 Impotence (erectile dysfunction)

Refer to the separate Chapter on impotence (erectile dysfunction).

6 Co-drivers (artificial insemination, IVF, etc)

Introduction

1 The term artificial insemination sounds daunting and cold. Some fertility clinics call it intra-uterine insemination for this very reason. Whatever it is called, it is actually a simple way of becoming pregnant if it is very difficult or impossible to manage it through sexual intercourse. If that does not work, more sophisticated treatments are available.

2 Note that impotence (erectile dysfunction/ED) and infertility are not the same thing. A man can be unable to have an erection yet be perfectly capable of having children by treating the erectile dysfunction (see *Impotence*) or by using assisted methods of conception. Sub-fertility, where there are too few sperm in the semen, or they are not able to swim correctly, does not necessarily mean that you cannot have children.

3 In cases of erectile dysfunction, seminal fluid can often be obtained by masturbation or by massaging the prostate under an anaesthetic. This is called AIP (artificial insemination by partner). With reduced fertility (sub-fertility) pregnancy can sometimes be achieved by placing the semen directly into the cervix. With severely reduced fertility, semen can be provided by another man. This is called AID (artificial insemination by donor). Most donors remain anonymous although the law is being pressed on this issue should your child wish to know their 'natural' father. You need to discuss this fully with your partner and medical staff.

4 Of course any form of artificial insemination carries connotations and must always be second best, but it is relatively easy, quick and results in the vast majority of cases in a perfectly normal baby.

Is there a problem?

5 Out of every ten couples trying for children eight achieve pregnancy within a year, one couple will conceive within two years and the remaining couple will need medical help. Many doctors will not consider referring a couple for infertility investigations until they have been trying for around two years (one year if the couple are over 35 years old).

6 How long you should spend trying for pregnancy before seeking help depends to some extent on the medical histories and age of you and your partner. Consult your GP or attend a family planning clinic for women if your partner:

- Has irregular periods, or the menstrual cycle is shorter than 21 or longer than 35 days.
- Finds intercourse painful.
- Has a history of pelvic inflammatory disease.

Dear Doctor

I've been going out with this lad for 14 months now. After the first four months of being together, we decided to get engaged and we decided to try for a baby but my fiancée has got premature ejaculation and I'm wondering is this the reason I'm not getting pregnant? This caused deep depression which caused me not to eat for months. I lost one and a half stones but slowly gained it again. My fiancée went to his local GP but was not happy. He gave him tablets and said call back. Desperately in need of any tips.

Premature ejaculation and delayed ejaculation are actually part of the same spectrum. It can be argued that there is no such thing as premature ejaculation as it by definition simply means reaching a climax too soon. The 'too soon' in this case is presumably before you have reached your own orgasm. So long as his penis is inside your vagina it actually makes no difference whether he reaches his climax early or late when it comes to having children. Premature ejaculation simply restricts the amount of pleasure experienced by both partners but particularly the woman. Medicines are not the answer. You can help prevent premature ejaculation by squeezing quite firmly at the base of the glans each time he feels he is about to climax. Both of you should ask to be referred to your local fertility clinic by your GP. It is possible that you are trying 'too hard'. The testes produce sperm at a more or less constant rate and if you have intercourse too often you will actually reduce the chance of becoming pregnant. Once a month is better than once per hour. Unfortunately this does tend to affect the fun side of the whole thing.

9

- Has had any abdominal surgery.
- Has a history of chlamydia or another sexually transmitted infection.
- Is underweight or overweight.
- Is aged over 35.

7 Consult your GP or attend a family planning clinic for men if you:

- Have had an operation on the testes, or had treatment for testicular cancer or an undescended testicle.
- Have a history of chlamydia or another sexually transmitted infection.
- Have a history of mumps after puberty.
- Are very overweight.

8 Be prepared to discuss questions such as:

- Your general medical health.
- Your partner's menstrual cycle.
- Previous methods of contraception.

- Any previous pregnancies/miscarriages/abortions.
- Any infections, including sexually transmitted infections.
- How often you have intercourse.

Causes of infertility and possible treatments

9 A woman who has difficulty in ovulating may need a course of drugs.

10 A woman not producing eggs may need another woman to donate eggs (this is not routinely offered).

11 A woman with blocked fallopian tubes may need surgery or assisted conception.

12 A man with a low count and/or poor quality of sperm may need assisted conception to aid fertilisation using his own sperm. Alternatively, sperm from a donor may be needed.

13 There may be other, less common, causes and a couple may have a combination of problems, so investigations need to be completed even if one problem is found at an early stage. Most problems can be helped, with varying degrees of success. Sometimes, even after full investigations, the reason for infertility cannot be found but assisted conception treatment may still be successful.

14 Visiting your GP gives you and your partner the opportunity to ask about the possible investigations and treatments, waiting lists and any costs. You can then decide if you want to go ahead with tests and/or treatment. You will want to know what treatments are offered locally on the NHS and, if you wish to consider paying for private treatment, what private treatments are available locally. You should also find out whether the NHS will meet the costs of any prescribed drugs or if you will have to pay for them.

15 While GPs can do some preliminary investigations, you may need to be referred to a specialist fertility clinic. If so, you will need a referral letter from your GP. The provision of specialist services within the NHS is limited in some areas and waiting lists vary for certain types of treatment, so try to find out how long you are likely have to wait for an appointment.

Eligibility for NHS treatment

16 The type of treatment you can receive on the NHS depends on a number of factors, including what infertility services local health services decide they will purchase.

17 Some patients will be investigated and treated at their local hospital, others may be referred on to a specialist unit. There is often a

Dear Doctor

I hope you can reassure me. I love my boyfriend very much but I recently discovered that he only has one testicle. He told me he lost one in an accident when he was little. We are talking about getting married and I want to have children. Will he still be able to father babies or will I have to use donor sperm? I know this sounds awfully selfish but I really don't want to do this and I am badly torn about still seeing him. Please help as I do love him although I'm sure you think I'm terrible.

No. You are not terrible. You are simply confused and badly informed. Millions of sperm are produced by each testis and it only takes one to fertilise the egg. Obviously the higher the sperm count the better the chance of a single sperm successfully making the long journey. Below a certain number, a man becomes sub-fertile but can still be a father although it may be necessary to give the sperm a 'helping hand' by placing them closer to where they are needed. Your boyfriend may simply have an undescended testicle. He should make sure that the one which failed to arrive on time has been removed, as there is a significantly increased chance of testicular cancer otherwise. Being honest with him about your concerns is the best policy. Your GP can help.

limit on the amount of treatment you can receive.

18 While most tests and investigations are carried out on the NHS, around 80 per cent of in-vitro fertilisation (IVF) treatment is carried out privately. You need to find out what the funding and selection criteria are to see if you will be eligible for NHS treatment. You could also contact the Human Fertilisation and Embryology Authority (HFEA) for a copy of its Patients' Guide to clinics. The reputations and success rates of different fertility clinics vary widely. If venturing outside the NHS, be wary of fraudulent practitioners – check on the HFEA website (see below).

Fertility tests

19 A specialist clinic will be able to carry out many different kinds of tests to see what the problem is and to find out which treatments will be best for you.

20 Clinics offer different types of treatment, and no single clinic is going to be best for everyone. Practical factors such as the opening times, the costs, the length of the clinic's waiting list and the travelling involved are also important.

21 The kind of tests that are done vary from clinic to clinic. Once you have a diagnosis, fairly simple treatment or surgery may be all that is needed. Not all of the following tests may be necessary, but they include:

- **Semen analysis** to look at the number, shape and size of sperm and how well they move. More than one test should be carried out.
- **Blood or urine tests** to check hormone levels.

- **X-rays/scans** to find blockages or check blood supply to the testes.
- **Blood, urine and cervical mucus checks** to verify hormone levels or detect ovulation.
- **Ultrasound scans** to check if a follicle, which should contain an egg, is being produced. Treatment for ovulation problems usually involves drugs by tablets, injections or nasal inhalations – and has a high success rate if the correct diagnosis has been established.
- **Sperm mucus crossover** – this checks if the woman's cervical mucus allows her partner's sperm through.
- **Endometrial biopsy** – a tiny sample of womb lining (endometrium) is removed to check that it is free from infection and that ovulation has occurred.
- **Hysterosalpingogram** where dye is passed through the fallopian tubes to check that they are open and clear of obstruction.
- **Laparoscopy** (usually under general anaesthetic) uses a thin telescope-like instrument to view the female reproductive organs through a small cut below the navel. It checks for scar tissue, endometriosis, fibroids or any abnormality in the shape or position of the womb, ovaries or fallopian tubes. At the same time a dye may be passed through the fallopian tubes to see if they are open and clear.

Assisted conception

22 Assisted conception techniques have been used successfully for many years and a range of techniques is available. It is now possible for some men with very low sperm counts or even with no sperm in their semen to have their own

genetic children. A specialist clinic will be able to advise you on which treatment will be best for you.

23 The most well-known treatment is in-vitro fertilisation (IVF) in which eggs are removed from the woman, fertilised in the laboratory and the embryo is then placed into her womb. Others include:

- **Donor Insemination (DI)** uses sperm from anonymous donor, where there are severe problems with the man's sperm.
- **Gamete Intra-Fallopian Transfer (GIFT)** uses a couple's own eggs and sperm, or those of donors, which are mixed together and placed in the woman's fallopian tubes where they fertilise.
- **Intra-Cytoplasmic Sperm Injection (ICSI)** uses a single sperm injected into the woman's egg which is then transferred to the womb after fertilisation.

24 These are not miracle solutions. The age of your partner is very important. A woman aged under 35 has a much better chance of a successful pregnancy than one over 40.

Donor insemination (DI) of sperm and donor eggs

25 If a man produces no or few normal sperm, carries an inherited disease, or has had a vasectomy, then insemination using sperm from an anonymous donor may be considered. Egg donation may be an option if a woman is not producing eggs or has a genetic problem. The decision to use donor sperm or eggs can be a difficult one. You can get help in making this decision from a counsellor or support group.

26 Clinics which offer this service have to send information about donors, recipients and the outcome of treatment to the HFEA. Donors have to meet extensive screening criteria, including HIV testing. A man may not usually donate sperm after ten live births have resulted from his semen donations. Donors do not have to be anonymous and most clinics will accept a donor who a couple have found for themselves.

Counselling and support

27 Couples report that the many hospital visits needed and the time spent waiting between treatments to learn if each stage has worked is stressful. All units providing IVF and other licensed conception techniques have a legal responsibility to offer counselling. Counselling can allow you to talk through what the treatment entails and how you feel about it, and can give support during the process and if the treatment fails.

28 If you don't want to see a counsellor at the clinic you are attending, the British Infertility Counsellors Association can put you in touch with your nearest infertility counsellor. Some people find being in contact with others in a similar situation or with a support group helps them through infertility.

Further information

29 If you would like to know more, look in the Contacts section at the back of the book, or contact:

Donor Conception Network
Tel 0208 245 4369
ww.dcnetwork.org
ISSUE: The National Fertility Association
Tel 09050 280 300 (25p/min)
ww.issue.co.uk

CHILD: The National Infertility Support Network
Tel 01424 732 361
www.child.org.uk

Human Fertilisation and Embryology Authority (HFEA)
Tel 020 7377 5077
Mon-Fri 9.30am-5.30pm
www.hfea.gov.uk

British Infertility Counsellors Association
Tel 0114 263 1448
www.bica.net

---

7 One or two car family?

Introduction

1 There are numerous methods of contraception, most of which, it has to be said, depend more on the woman than the man. Not only is there a difference in the way the methods work and are used, but there is a significant difference in the protection each method provides.

The male condom

2 Society is increasingly accepting the condom as one of the normal requirements of modern life. This has led to their wider availability and condoms can now readily be obtained – in supermarkets, from garages, by mail order, through slot machines, as well as in pharmacies. They are free from all family planning clinics and genito-urinary medicine clinics. Colours, flavours and new materials, like plastic, make interesting options. Condoms now come in different shapes and sizes, and it is often necessary to try a few different types before the right one is found. If used correctly condoms are 98 per cent effective at preventing pregnancy and they have the added advantage of providing good protection against many sexually transmitted infections. Hermetically sealed, the modern condom will remain usable for a long time (look for the expiry date); good quality condoms will also have the CE mark and the kitemark. Once the seal is broken they should be used quite soon as the rubber will perish on exposure to the air and the lubricant will dry, making it difficult to put on.

Use of condoms

3 Using a condom correctly is essential for it to be effective. It should be put on before any contact between the penis and the vagina or genital area, and rolled on the correct way round. Air should be excluded from the end of the condom as it can cause it to burst or slip off. Sharp finger nails, rings and teeth are a hazard. Only the soft

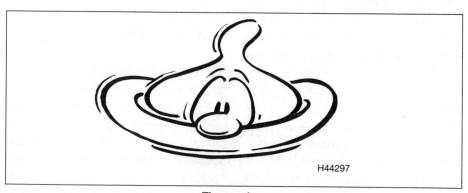

H44297

The condom

finger pulps should be used to unroll the condom on to the penis. If extra lubrication is needed then only a water based one should be used with rubber condoms. There is a need to withdraw and remove the condom while the penis is still erect to avoid semen leaking out as the penis shrinks in size.

Spontaneity

4 Perhaps the single biggest stated reason for not using condoms is the widely held belief that they inhibit spontaneous sex. Foreplay is an important part of enjoyable sexual activity and partners can involve the condom in this. Fears that they reduce the sensitivity of sexual experience have not been supported by research. Most of the problem is with the psychological inhibition some men have over their use but without doubt lots of foreplay does help.

The female condom

5 The condom for women is relatively new, but regular users report favourably and many men prefer them to the male condom. Made of plastic it is larger in diameter than the male condom and has a flexible ring at each end. The smaller ring fits inside the vagina while the outer, larger, ring remains on the outside of the vagina. After ejaculation this outer ring should be twisted to prevent escape of the sperm and the condom gently withdrawn. Female condoms are 95 per cent effective, and also have the advantage of providing protection against many sexually transmitted infections.

Oral contraception (the Pill)

6 The combined pill contains two hormones which inhibit the release of the hormones which stimulate the final development and release of ova (eggs) from the ovary. This partly mimics a pregnancy, which explains why some women suffer the milder symptoms of being pregnant when using this pill.

7 The combined pill is convenient, over 99 per cent effective when taken correctly, and has many advantages (including protection against cancer of the womb and the ovary). Like all drugs, there are health risks associated with its use. A very small number of women will develop a blood clot which can be life-threatening. Women who take the pill are also more at risk of being diagnosed with breast cancer or cervical cancer. However, for the vast majority of women the advantages of taking the pill greatly outweigh the risks.

8 The progestogen-only pill contains only one hormone and stops sperm from getting anywhere near the egg by maintaining the natural plug of mucus in the neck of the womb. It also makes the lining of the womb thinner. It is highly effective (99 per cent) and it is particularly useful for women who cannot use the combined pill, and those who are breast-feeding. It has, however, to be taken regularly at the same time each day, and can have the disadvantage of causing irregular bleeding.

Intrauterine contraceptive device (IUD)

9 These small plastic and copper devices are inserted into the womb by GPs, or by doctors or nurses at family planning clinics. They prevent pregnancy by stopping the sperm and egg meeting; they also make the lining of the womb unsuitable for implantation should fertilisation occur. They are over 99 per cent effective, can be left in place for up to eight years, and can be used by women both before and after having children. They are not suitable for women who are at risk of getting a sexually transmitted infection, and can make periods longer and heavier. To minimise the risk of infection, tests are done before the IUD is put in. The IUD is removed very easily by a doctor or nurse and has no effect upon sensation during intercourse.

Intrauterine contraceptive system (IUS)

10 These small plastic T shaped devices contain the hormone progestogen. They are inserted into the womb by GPs, or by doctors or nurses at family planning clinics. They prevent pregnancy in the same way as the progestogen-only pill. They are over 99 per cent effective, can be left in place for up to five years, and can be used by women both before and after having children. Initial side-effects can include irregular bleeding, but periods then tend to become lighter and shorter, or stop altogether; period pain is also reduced. Like the IUD, the IUS is removed very easily by a doctor or nurse and has no effect upon sensation during intercourse.

Hormone implant (for women)

11 One small rod containing progestogen is inserted under the skin in the arm, usually using a local anaesthetic. It works like the progestogen-only pill and lasts for three years. The main disadvantage is that it can cause irregular bleeding for several months. It is over 99 per cent effective and is easily removed in a minute or two.

9

CONTRACEPTIVE METHODS WITH POSSIBILITY OF USER FAILURE

The methods in this table must be used correctly to achieve the effectiveness stated.

	Combined pill	Progestogen-only pill	Male condom	Female condom	Diaphragm or cap	Natural family planning (NFP)
How it works	Contains two hormones, oestrogen and progestogen, which stop ovulation.	Contains the hormone progestogen, which thickens the cervical mucus, and stops sperm getting near the egg.	Barrier method. The condom covers the penis and stops sperm entering the vagina.	Barrier method. The condom lines the vagina and stops sperm entering.	Barrier method. A rubber or silicone cap covers the cervix to keep sperm out of the womb. Used with spermicidal cream or jelly.	Fertile and infertile times in the menstrual cycle are identified.
Pros	Can reduce PMS, period pain and bleeding. Protects against cancer of the womb and ovary.	Can be used when breast-feeding. More suitable for older smokers than the combined pill.	Wide choice and easy availability. Provides some protection against sexually transmitted infections. Under male control.	Can be put in before sex. Provides some protection against sexually transmitted infections.	Can be put in before sex. Provides some protection against sexually transmitted infections.	Freedom from side-effects. Awareness of fertile times can be used for planning pregnancies as well as avoiding them.
Cons	Increased risk of breast and cervical cancer. Increased risk of thrombosis (blood clots).	May produce irregular periods with bleeding in between. May be less effective in women weighing over 70 kg (11 stone).	Need to stop to put it on. Can split or come off if not used correctly. Need to withdraw while still erect.	If not inserted in advance, need to stop to put it in. Need to make sure that the penis enters correctly.	If not inserted in advance, need to stop to put it in. Can provoke cystitis in some users.	Method must be taught by a qualified teacher. Users must abstain from sex, or use a barrier method, during the fertile period.
Remarks	Smokers over 35 should not use it (risk of thrombosis).	Must be taken at exactly the same time each day (to within 3 hours).	Do not re-use. Must be put on before genital contact occurs. Do not use oil-based lubricants on latex condoms.	Do not re-use. Must be put in before genital contact occurs. Expensive to buy, but can be obtained free at some family planning clinics.	Must be correctly fitted, and fit must be checked every 12 months. Must be put in before genital contact occurs.	There are various different methods of indicating fertility. Effectiveness is highest when using several indicators.
Effectiveness*	Over 99%	99%	98%	95%	92% to 96%	Up to 98%

* Effectiveness is expressed as the percentage of women who will not get pregnant with each year of correct use of a particular contraceptive method. So if the effectiveness is 99%, 1 woman in 100 will get pregnant in a year. Using no contraception at all, 80 to 90 women out of 100 will get pregnant in a year.

CONTRACEPTIVE METHODS WITH NO POSSIBILITY OF USER FAILURE

The effectiveness of the methods in this table does not depend on the user.

	Contraceptive injection	Implant	Intrauterine system (IUS)	Intrauterine device (IUD)	Female sterilisation	Male sterilisation (vasectomy)
How it works	The hormone progestogen is slowly released, stopping ovulation and thickening the cervical mucus.	An implant is placed under the skin. It releases the hormone progestogen, stopping ovulation and thickening the cervical mucus.	A small plastic device is inserted into the womb. It releases the hormone progestogen, thickening the cervical mucus.	A small plastic and copper device is inserted into the womb. It stops sperm meeting an egg, or fertilised eggs implanting.	The fallopian tubes are cut, sealed or otherwise blocked. The egg cannot meet the sperm.	The tubes carrying the sperm from each testis are cut or blocked. There are no sperm in the semen.
Pros	Single injection lasts for 8 or 12 weeks. Protects against cancer of the womb and ovary.	Single implant works for 3 years. Quickly reversed at any time.	Single insertion lasts for 5 years. Quickly reversed at any time. Periods are normally lighter and less painful.	Single insertion lasts for up to 10 years (depending on model). Effective immediately.	Permanent. No known long-term side-effects.	Permanent. No known long-term side-effects. Minor operation under local anaesthetic.
Cons	Fertility may take a year to return after stopping the injections. Periods may become irregular or stop. Other side-effects, including weight gain, in some users.	Periods may become irregular or stop. Other side-effects, including weight gain, in some users.	Irregular light bleeding for the first 3 months is common; sometimes this lasts longer. Other side-effects in some users.	Periods may become, heavier, longer and more painful. Not suitable for women at risk of catching a sexually transmitted infection.	Invasive surgical procedure under general anaesthetic. Small possibility (1 in 200) of tubes rejoining and restoring fertility.	Expect some swelling and discomfort after the operation. Very small possibility (1 in 2000) of tubes rejoining.
Remarks	Effects cannot be stopped until the injection runs out.	Usually inserted and removed using a local anaesthetic.	Useful for women with very heavy or painful periods.	IUD insertion can also be used as emergency contraception.	Should be assumed to be irreversible. Other contraception must be used until the first period after sterilisation.	Should be assumed to be irreversible. Other contraception must be used until there have been two consecutive negative sperm tests.
Effectiveness*	Over 99%	Over 99%	Over 99%	98% or better	99.5%	99.95%

* Effectiveness is expressed as the percentage of women who will not get pregnant with each year of correct use of a particular contraceptive method. So if the effectiveness is 99%, 1 woman in 100 will get pregnant in a year. Using no contraception at all, 80 to 90 women out of 100 will get pregnant in a year.

1

Hormone injection (for women)

12 The hormone progestogen is given as an injection every 8 or 12 weeks, depending on the type used. It is over 99 per cent effective and works by stopping the ovaries producing eggs. It shares many of the advantages of the combined pill, but can cause irregular bleeding and weight gain. Once the injections stop it can take a year or more for periods to return.

The male Pill

13 The day when a male pill will be available slowly gets nearer. There have been successful human trials in the UK, and in the next decade we should see a male hormonal method of contraception. At the moment it is unclear whether this will be in the form of a pill, an implant or an injection.

Female sterilisation

14 This is a permanent method of contraception in which the fallopian tubes are either cut, sealed or blocked so that eggs cannot pass down them to the uterus (womb). It has a failure rate of 1 in 200, making it 99.5 per cent effective – as good as other long-term reversible methods. Should it fail, it carries a greater risk of the egg implanting in the fallopian tube (ectopic pregnancy). As a general anaesthetic is required and the operation is more invasive it is a more complicated and risky procedure than vasectomy. It is possible to reverse the operation but with limited success, and with an increased risk of ectopic pregnancy.

Emergency contraception

15 'Emergency' contraception is a safe and effective way of preventing pregnancy. It involves either taking tablets containing progestogen (which are used within 72 hours of sex but are more effective the sooner they are taken) or inserting an IUD. Emergency methods can be used when no contraception was used or when regular contraception has failed. Emergency pills are safe to take and have no lasting effects on future fertility. Emergency contraception is available free from GPs, family planning clinics. In addition emergency pills are free from NHS Walk-in centres and can be bought from pharmacies by women over 16.

Natural methods

16 It is only possible for your partner to conceive within 24 hours of ovulation. However, because sperm can live for several days, sex that happens up to seven days before ovulation can result in pregnancy (this sex can even be during a period). It is possible to estimate the fertile period by noting certain changes in the body. Using a fertility thermometer and a chart it is possible to detect the sudden rise in temperature of around 0.2 degrees Celsius which occurs at ovulation. Monitoring changes in the cervical mucus help identify the time before and after ovulation. The mucus becomes thin, watery and clearer before ovulation, and afterwards returns to being thicker, stickier and whiter. When practised according to instruction, natural family planning is 98 per cent effective, although it does take a while to learn it as a method and requires commitment from both partners.

Vasectomy (male sterilisation)

17 Vasectomy is a simple and permanent method of contraception. You don't need permission from your partner but obviously it makes good sense. Fortunately there is no reported effect on enjoying sex. The

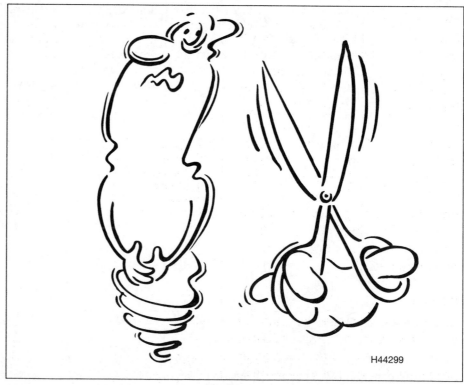

H44299

Vasectomy

testicles continue to produce sperm but rather than being ejaculated with the semen the sperm are reabsorbed in each testicle. Sperm therefore doesn't build up inside the testicles. As with any surgical procedure you will have to sign a consent form.

When it should be done

18 Although there is no lower age limit for vasectomy, young, childless men need to consider this method carefully to avoid later regret. It should therefore only be chosen by men who, for whatever reason, are sure that they do not want children in the future. Counselling is recommended so that other contraception options can be discussed and the procedure fully understood. A vasectomy immediately following a birth, miscarriage, abortion or family or relationship crisis is a usually a bad idea.

How it is performed

19 You can ask for a general anaesthetic but it is generally performed under a local anaesthetic. A small section of each vas deferens – the tubes carrying the sperm from the testes – is removed through small cuts on either side of the scrotum **(see illustration)**. The ends of the tubes are then cut or blocked. Stitches are rarely required on the scrotum. It is a simple and safe operation lasting around 10-15 minutes, and can be done in a clinic, hospital outpatient department or doctor's surgery.

Recovery

20 Discomfort and swelling lasting for a few days is normal but this settles quickly with no other problems. Simple pain-killers help. Occasionally this can last longer and needs your doctor's attention. Strenuous activity should be avoided for a week but you can return to work immediately and have sex as soon as it is comfortable. As the testicles continue to produce testosterone your feelings, sex drive, ability to have an erection and climax won't be affected. Despite numerous scares in the popular media, there are no known long-term risks from a vasectomy.

Effectiveness

21 After a vasectomy it can take a few months for all the sperm to disappear from your semen. You need to use another method of contraception until you have had two consecutive semen tests which show that you have no sperm. While vasectomy is highly effective failures are still possible (1 in 2000). The failure rate should be discussed before the operation and it should be pointed out on the consent form. While vasectomy is excellent in preventing pregnancy it will not protect against sexually-transmitted infections. Using a condom is the best protection for this.

Future prospects

22 Reversal operations are possible but not always successful and will depend upon how and when the vasectomy was done. Reversals are not easily available either privately or on the NHS.

Further information

23 If you would like to know more, look in the Contacts section at the back of the book, or contact:

Sexual Health Direct (run by The Family Planning Association)
Tel 0845 310 1334
Mon-Fri 9am-7pm
www.fpa.org.uk

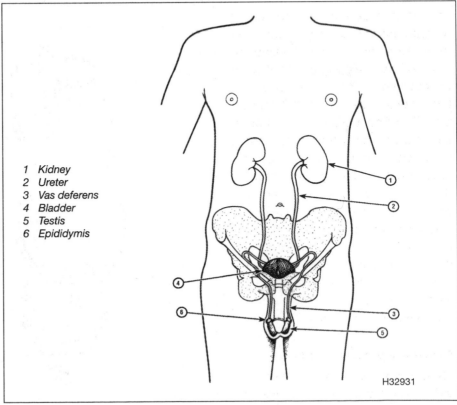

1 Kidney
2 Ureter
3 Vas deferens
4 Bladder
5 Testis
6 Epididymis

H32931

The male urogenital system

9

Chapter 10
Impotence (erectile dysfunction)

Contents

1 Introduction

1 Even in these enlightened times there is still confusion over erectile dysfunction (ED/impotence) and infertility. A man can father children without being able to have an erection. Problems with erections are common. At least one in 10 British men have had some sort of erectile dysfunction at some stage in their lives. Furthermore, around one man in twenty has permanent erectile dysfunction problems. This is not helped by most men's reluctance to discuss these problems, despite the fact that virtually all of them can be overcome by relatively simple treatments.

2 As the penis works by hydrostatic pressure allowing blood into the spongy tissues of the penis but restricting its outflow, anything which affects the blood vessels or nerves which bring this about will influence the ability to have an erection. Unfortunately there are a large number of things which will interfere with this process, not least medicines prescribed for totally different reasons.

3 At one time, what was going on between a man's ears was considered the major factor for ED. We now know that around one third of all cases will be purely psychological, and will often respond well to non-clinical treatments such as sex counselling. Generally speaking, if you have erections at any other time other than during attempted intercourse then you have a psychological rather than physiological problem. Successful erections during television programmes, sexy videos or self-masturbation bode well for the future, although it is not a 100 per cent test.

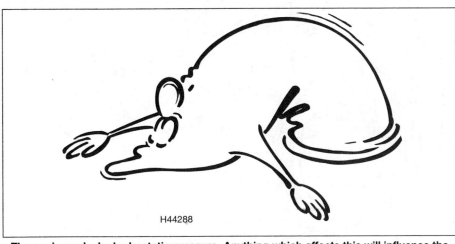

H44288

The penis works by hydrostatic pressure. Anything which affects this will influence the ability to have an erection

Dear Doctor

I've heard about patches for men to help with impotence. My doctor already gives me hormone replacement therapy. My husband has problems sometimes getting an erection. Unfortunately he has to pay for his prescriptions. Can he use my patches instead and save the money?

Your husband can certainly use your patches. He may find however that will also have to use your Wonderbra. Hormone replacement for women involves the use of the female sex hormone oestrogen. While it most definitely is useful at preventing thin bones in women, it does nothing for a man in a wet sweatshirt. The male equivalent uses testosterone, the male sex hormone. It can help with impotence but only if the problem is caused by a lack of the hormone in the first place.

2 When the flesh needs convincing

1 While there is great variation in the actual size of the penis throughout the animal kingdom, humans come top of the list in their group, the primates. (However, unlike some of the other primates we do not have prehensile tails.) For all primates the penis appears to have a disproportionate influence over the everyday life of the species; few other animals give sex, as distinct from reproduction, the same level of priority. Similarly, the role of the human penis is complex and extends beyond a means of transferring sperm to the female or even passing urine. Society places a certain importance on the size of a man's penis. It is said that the CIA seriously considered supplying over-sized condoms to villagers during the Vietnam/Cambodian war to enhance the 'prowess' of American troops in the eyes of the enemy.

Hydraulic system

2 There is no bone in the penis. Its function depends upon a hydraulic system which Citroën owners will readily understand. Just as a balloon filled with water is more rigid than one without, the erect penis uses the same principle, using blood rather than water as the stiffening medium. By allowing blood into spongy tissue within the penis, but restricting its exit, the penis can enlarge by around 2 inches during an erection.

3 While valuable for placing sperm well into the vagina, an erection hinders the passing of urine. Indeed there is a one-way valve at the base of the penis which prevents urine being passed at the same time as sperm. Urine or sperm travel down the penis from the bladder or testes in a thin tube called the urethra.

4 The thin skin of the penis is covered in small bumps which may be important in stimulation of the sexual partner. Unfortunately they also cause a disproportionate amount of concern, particularly amongst young men. These are the sweat glands and hair follicles that are not normally felt on thicker skin. They are even more noticeable during an erection because the skin is stretched much thinner.

Average sizes

5 While men are prone to exaggerate, the average size of the human penis is around three-and-a-half to seven inches. There are

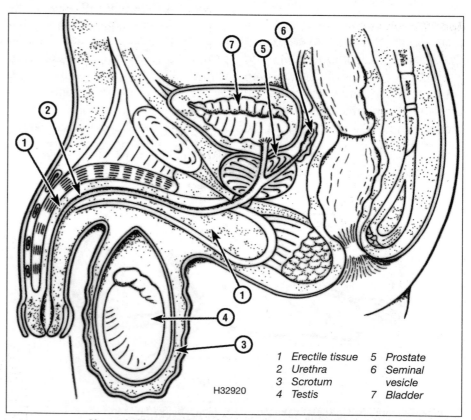

H32920

1 Erectile tissue	5 Prostate
2 Urethra	6 Seminal
3 Scrotum	vesicle
4 Testis	7 Bladder

Almost half the penile structure is hidden within the pelvis

operations which lengthen the penis by up to 50 per cent as almost half the penile structure is hidden within the pelvis. By cutting the ligaments which tether the penis to the pubic bones, the true length is exposed. The only serious side effect is the alteration in the angle of dangle. Instead of the erect penis standing to attention, it tends to take a more horizontal position. This is not said to adversely affect sexual pleasure. Numerous studies, however, have shown that penile length is not the main factor for sexual pleasure in the female or male partner.

6 A more effective and far less traumatic way of increasing penis length is to lose any excess weight.

3 Erectile Dysfunction (ED)

Age: the great escape

1 If ever there was a universal scapegoat for things that go wrong with the human body, particularly sexual activity, it has to be 'too many birthdays'. Thankfully we are realising that sex is not just for the young and the enjoyment of sex can go on indefinitely. Expressions such as 'dirty old man' are becoming less common as we all live longer and older people predominate in our society.

2 Age-related problems do exist, but they are by no mean the major cause. Some important facts have emerged with recent studies:

* There is a gradual decline in testosterone levels and levels of this hormone can have an effect on target organs such as the penis.
* Erections take longer to develop and may require more tactile stimulation. Yes, the old Bentley may take longer to start than the new Porsche but it will give you a more comfortable ride. Might not run out of petrol so soon either.
* Self image and concerns over sexual activity tend to be problems in later life. Men are notoriously bad at confronting these problems and will often let age take the blame.
* Physical illnesses take their toll on sexual activity, not least because of the drugs which are commonly prescribed by way of treatment. We do tend to accumulate chronic conditions as we age.
* Gaps in sexual activity can be important, if only the toll they can take on sexual confidence. Bereavement, illness of the partner or divorce are good examples.
* Men are slow to admit depression to their doctors, older men even more so. Depression is a major factor for erectile dysfunction.

Common medicines and alcohol

3 Some medicines are known to cause problems with erections:

* Some anti-depressants are paradoxically capable of making erectile dysfunction even worse.

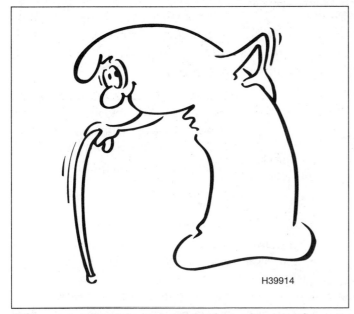

With age, erections take longer to develop and may require more tactile stimulation

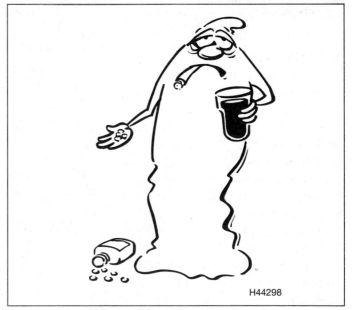

Medicines and alcohol can be a factor

On the other hand, some can delay premature ejaculation, which can be helpful. Talk to your doctor.

- Some anti-hypertensive drugs for high blood pressure are common culprits. ACE inhibitors, alpha and beta blockers, and calcium channel blockers can all cause problems for certain individuals. You can change your medicine to help. Talk to your doctor.
- Alcohol is a common cause. Obviously binge drinking has an immediate effect but chronic alcohol abuse can lead to permanent problems with erectile dysfunction. Small amounts of alcohol in the blood (up to 25 mg per 100 ml, or a couple of drinks in plain English) make erections easier. Any more can cause the dreaded 'droop'.
- Tobacco has an immediate short-term effect but is a much worse long-term factor. You can't have an erection when you're dead.

Common disease culprits

4 Diseases which affect the nerves or blood supply can also cause problems:

- Multiple sclerosis is the commonest spinal cord disease causing erectile dysfunction. There can also be bladder problems.
- Diabetes can cause a peripheral nerve problem which affects the ability to have an erection and tends to go undiagnosed for many years.
- Vascular (blood circulation) problems account for around 25 per cent of erectile dysfunction in men. They usually have an insidious onset and are made worse by taking even small amounts of alcohol.

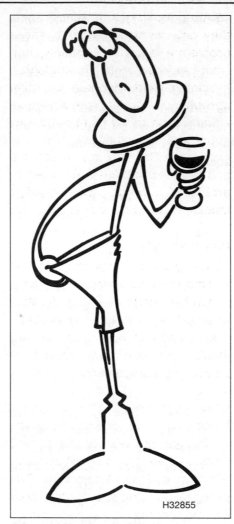

It is a golden opportunity to have a proper medical check for any underlying cause of erectile dysfunction

Diagnosis

5 A proper medical check-up is needed to look for any underlying cause of erectile dysfunction.

6 Your history will be the most important tool for diagnosis, but various tests on hormone levels are often performed.

7 Some diseases which travel in families, such as diabetes, hypertension or depression can also be an important clue to diagnosis. Details of drinking habits (remember brewer's droop?), smoking, diet and exercise can all be important.

Examination

8 A number of tests can be performed to exclude physiological causes. These include tests for:

- Diabetes.
- Anaemia.
- Liver problems.
- Thyroid deficiency (the thyroid is a gland in the neck which acts as a sort of thermostat for body metabolism. If it is set 'too low' then everything slows down, including erections).
- Testosterone, prolactin and leutenising hormone levels. The balance between all three show if you are producing the right levels of hormone to make erections possible in the first place.

9 Your doctor will also check:

- Blood circulation. Poor blood flow thorough arteries in your legs can also mean the same thing for your penis. Your legs use bone to stay straight, your penis can only use the pressure of blood.
- Loss of facial hair, large breasts or small testes. These all indicate a hormone problem.

Prevention

10 Avoiding excessive alcohol and tobacco are the obvious first lines of attack. Check with your doctor whether any drugs you are taking could be part of the problem.

Treatment

11 Herbal and traditional remedies are freely available but there is little evidence for their effectiveness.

12 Some simple treatments require a sense of humour, not least vacuum devices which have been around for over 70 years. They work by drawing blood into the penis under a gentle vacuum produced by a sheath placed over the penis and evacuated with a small pump. By restricting the blood from leaving with a tight rubber band at the base of the penis, a respectable erection can be produced. It makes sense to remove the band after 30 minutes or so to avoid problems with blood clotting. They can be used in men with vascular problems.

Psychological causes

13 The treatment of psychological impotence depends on education, the use of methods such as the temporary prohibition of sexual intercourse, the encouragement of touching and sensual massage (sensate focus technique) and sexual counselling.

14 You will need to be honest with yourself and your counsellor. They will want to know a number of important things:

- Childhood experiences and your attitude to sexuality. This may well include the attitudes of your partner.
- Your sexual experience during adolescence.
- Your own body image and how you feel about your genitals.
- How content you are with your sexual relationships.
- 'Bad trips'. Have you had some painful experiences which are flavouring your appreciation of sex.
- Your feelings about sexual arousal. What is 'normal' or 'acceptable' practice.
- How you rate yourself as a sexual being.

15 After looking into these areas they will want to know if these problems came on suddenly, and what preceded them. Psychological problems tend to come on quite abruptly whereas physiological causes tend to be more insidious. Your medical history will be examined. Some drugs (medicinal and recreational) can cause erectile problems. Even homeopathic treatments can be a factor.

Oral treatments

16 The great leap forward came with oral preparations which are increasing in number, mode of action, duration of action and safety. They allow as near as possible 'normal' sex but still require stimulation and arousal as they are not aphrodisiacs.

17 Although around 80% of men will be able to get an erection adequate for intercourse with drug support, probably less than half will continue with therapy in the longer term. The likely reason for this is that both doctors and their male patients tend to focus on erection and genital function rather than on sexual satisfaction, and this is a very personal factor. A rigid erection alone will not necessarily help you talk comfortably and openly about your sexual fantasies and ideas, particularly if you have not had sex for a long time.

18 Couples using drug therapies need ongoing support and encouragement until they are satisfied with the outcome of treatment. It is important that you understand how to use the drugs properly as nearly one third of men who failed to get adequate erections with a drug could do so when re-instructed on its proper use.

19 Another important issue is that, whether using drug therapy or not, older men take longer to get an erection and often require direct genital stimulation to do so. Some men believe that their inability to get an erection through fantasy or visual stimulation alone is abnormal, whereas it should really be expected with ageing. Variety really can be quite literally the spice of life here and more variety in sexual behaviour can be helpful. Cuddling, play and talking are all part of the sex act which will have gone as well so needs to be put back into practice.

Injections

20 Hormone injections straight into the penis may be a better option. The needle is so fine it is virtually painless but you need to inject into different places to stop any scarring.

21 Injections of drugs straight into the spongy tissue of the penis can mimic the way the nerves work by restricting the blood flow out of the penis, thus producing an erection in men with these problems. It is surprisingly free of pain, although most men cross their legs just thinking about it.

22 These treatments can be effective in men who have not responded to oral therapies, but they may not always be acceptable to men or their partners. Unlike oral therapies, they provoke erection directly without the need for external stimulation.

Penile implants

23 If there is no response to injections, a penile prosthesis may be the answer. Before you go down this road both you and your partner need to understand what is involved. There is a certain sacrifice of dignity which both of you will need to come to terms with. Having said that, many couples find the release of sexual frustration far outweighs the temporary embarrassment.

24 There are three versions of implantable devices:

- Semi-rigid rods, made of silicone, sometimes covered with stainless steel braiding, are inserted into the spongy tissue of the penis.
- Two self-contained cylinder pumps are inserted into the penis and filled by squeezing a reservoir in the base of the penis.
- Inflatable penis prostheses consist of a pair of inflatable silicone cylinders implanted in the penis which can be filled by squeezing a pump implanted in the scrotum.

25 They all work. But as the old saying goes, 'it's not the size, it's what you do with it that counts'. Foreplay, sexual experimentation, avoidance of routine and being honest with each other is just as important as having a functional erection. Oh yes, and a healthy dollop of a sense of humour too. Sex after all is not only enjoyable, it can be good fun as well.

Further information

26 If you would like to know more, look in the Contacts section at the back of the book, or contact:

Relate
www.relate.org.uk

Impotence Association
Tel 020 8757 7791
www.impotence.org.uk

Reference

Contents

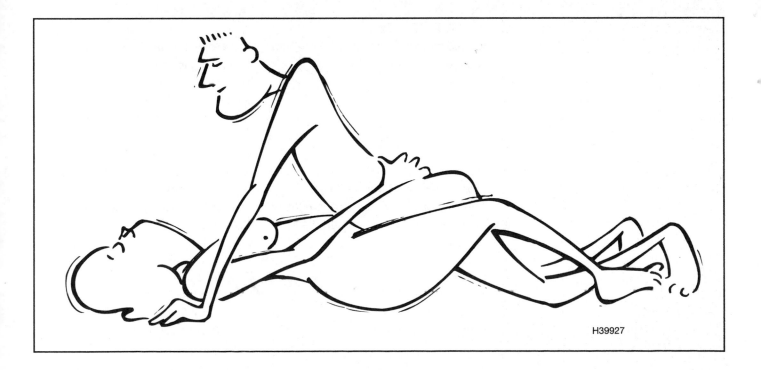

H39927

Contacts

Alcoholics Anonymous
PO Box 1
Stonebow House
Stonebow
York YO1 7NJ
Tel 01904 644026

Black HIV-AIDS Network Limited
St Stephens House
41 Uxbridge Road
London W12 8LH
Tel 020 8749 2828

Body Positive
51b Philbeach Gardens
Earls Court
London SW5 9EB
Tel 020 7835 1045

British Association for Sexual and
Relationship Therapy
PO Box 13686
London SW20 9ZH
www.basrt.org.uk

British Heart Foundation
14 Fitzhardinge Street
London W1H 6DH
020 7935 0185
www.bhf.org.uk

British Infertility Counselling
Association
69 Division Street
Sheffield
S1 4GE
Tel 0114 263 1448
www.bica.net

Cancer Research UK
PO Box 123
Lincoln's Inn Fields
London
WC2A 3PX
020 7009 8820
www.cancerresearchuk.org

CHILD: The National Infertility
Support Network
Tel 01424 732 361
www.child.org.uk

Community Hygiene Concern
Manor Gardens Centre
6-9 Manor Gardens
London N7 6LA
Tel 020 7686 4321
www.chc.org

Diabetes UK
10 Parkway
London NW1 7AA
Tel 020 7424 1030

Donor Conception Network
(For advice, information and support
on donor insemination)
PO Box 265
Sheffield S3 7YX
Tel 020 8245 4369
www.dcnetwork.org

Drinkline
(For advice and information on
reducing alcohol consumption)
Tel 0800 917 8282
www.downyourdrink.org/drinkline.html
www.wrecked.co.uk

Epilepsy Action
0808 800 5050
www.epilepsy.org.uk

Family Planning Association
(For advice and information on
contraception, sexually transmitted
infections and other sexual health
issues)
2-12 Pentonville Road
London N1 9FP
Mon-Fri 9am-7pm
Tel 0845 310 1334
www.fpa.org.uk

Human Fertilisation and Embryology
Authority (HFEA)
Mon-Fri 9.30am-5.30pm
Tel 020 7377 5077
www.hfea.gov.uk

Impotence Association
(For information and advice on all
sexual dysfunctions)
PO Box 10296
London SW17 9WH
Tel 020 8767 7791
www.impotence.org.uk

International Stress Management
Association
The Priory Hospital, Priory Lane
London SW15 5JJ

ISSUE The National Fertility
Association
(Provides advice, information and
support on fertility problems.)
114 Lichfield Street
Walsall
West Midlands, WS1 1SZ
Tel 01922 722888
www.issue.co.uk

The Men's Health Forum
Tavistock House
Tavistock Square
London, WC1H 9HR
www.menshealthforum.org.uk

The Million Women Study
A national study of women's health
Professor Valerie Beal
The Million Women Study
Co-ordinating Centre
Cancer Research UK,
Epidemiological Unit
Gibson Building
Radcliffe Infirmary
Oxford, OX2 6HE
www.millionwomenstudy.org.uk

MIND (National Association For Mental Health)
Granta House
15-19 Broadway
Stratford
London
E15 4BQ

National Action on Incontinence (Incontact)
Mon-Fri 9am-6pm
Tel 0191 213 0050

The National AIDS Helpline
Tel 0800 567 123 (English, Chinese and Cantonese)
Tel 0800 282 445 (English, Bengali, Hindu, Punjabi and Urdu)
www.playingsafely.co.uk

National Childbirth Trust
(For information on ante-natal classes, childbirth and local groups for parents/fathers)
Alexandra House Oldham Terrace
London
W3 6NH
Tel 0870 444 8707
www.nct-online.org

National Council for One Parent Families
(Founded in 1918, a national charity working to promote the interests of lone parents and their children and at the forefront of change to improve their lives)
255 Kentish Town Road
London
NW5 2LX
Tel 0800 018 5026
www.oneparentfamilies.org.uk

National Osteoporosis Society
Tel 01761 471771
www.nos.org.uk

NHS Direct
An online health information service (includes child health)
Tel 0845 4647
www.nhsdirect.nhs.uk

NORM-UK
www.norm-uk.org

The Orchid Cancer Appeal
St Bartholomews Hospital
London, EC1A 7BE
www.orchid-cancer.org.uk
info@orchid-cancer.org.uk

The Prostate Cancer Charity
3 Angel Walk, Hammersmith
London W6 9HX
Tel 0845 300 8383
www.prostate-cancer.org.uk

Prostate Help Association
Langworth , Lincoln LN3 5DF

Prostate Research Campaign UK
Canada House
272 Field End Road
Eastcote
Middlesex HA4 9NA
020 8582 0246
www.prostate-research.org.uk
info@prostate-research.org.uk

QUIT
Ground Floor
211 Old Street
London EC1V 9NR

Smokers' Quit-line
0800 00 22 00
www.quit.org.uk

Relate
(For counselling for relationship and/or sexual problems)
Tel 0845 1304010
www.relate.org.uk

Rethink (previously the NSF)
Head Office
30 Tabernacle Street
London EC2A 4DD
Tel 020 7330 9100
www.rethink.org

Samaritans
(For emotional support for people in crisis or at risk of suicide)
General Office
10 The Grove
Slough
Berks
SL1 1QP
Tel 08457 90 90 90
www.samaritans.org

Sex Education Forum
(Provides information and guidance to parents)
Tel 020 7843 6052
www.ncb.org.uk/sef/index.htm

Sexual Health Direct (Run by the Family Planning Association)
Mon-Fri 9am-7pm
Tel 0845 310 1334
www.fpa.org.uk

The Terrence Higgins Trust
(For advice and information on HIV and AIDS)
52-54 Grays Inn Road
London
WC1X 8JU
Monday-Friday 10am-10pm, Saturday-Sunday Noon-6pm
020 7242 1010
www.tht.org.uk

World Cancer Research Fund
19 Harley Street
London
W1G 9QJ
Tel 020 7343 4200
Web www.wcrf-uk.org

Further reading

Banks, Ian *Ask Dr Ian about Men's Health* (The Blackstaff Press, Belfast, 1997)

Banks, Ian *Ask Dr Ian About Sex* (The Blackstaff Press, Belfast, 1999)

Banks, Ian *Get Fit With Brittas* (BBC, 1998)

Banks, Ian *The Baby Manual* (Haynes Publishing, 2003)

Banks, Ian *The Dad's Survival Guide* (The Blackstaff Press, Belfast, 2001)

Banks, Ian *The Man Manual* (Haynes Publishing, 2002)

Banks, Ian *The NHS Direct Healthcare Guide* (Radcliffe Press, 2000)

Banks, Ian *The Trouble With Men* (BBC, 1997)

Baker, Peter *Real Health for Men* (Vega, 2002)

Beare, Helen and Priddy, Neil *The Cancer Guide for Men* (Sheldon Press, London, 1999)

Bechtel, Stefan and Stains, Laurence Roy *Sex: A Man's Guide* (Rodale Press, Emmaus)

Bradford, Nikki *Men's Health Matters: The Complete A-Z of Male Health* (Vermilion, London, 1995)

Brewer, Sarah *The Complete Book of Men's Health* (Thorsons, London, 1995)

Carroll, Steve *The Which? Guide to Men's Health* (Which?, London, 1999)

Cooper, Mick and Baker, Peter *The MANual: The Complete Man's Guide to Life* (Thorsons, London,1996)

Devlin, David and Webber, Christine *The Big O* (Hodder,1995)

Diagram Group, The *Man's Body: An Owner's Manual* (Wordsworth Editions, Ware, Hertfordshire, 1998)

Diamond, John *C: Because Cowards get Cancer too.* (Vermilion, London, 1999)

Egger, Garry *Trim For Life: 201 tips for effective weight control* (Allen & Unwin, St Leonards, Australia, 1997)

Gillie, Oliver *Regaining Potency: The answer to male impotence* (Self-Help Direct, London, 1997)

Goleman, Daniel *Emotional Intelligence: Why it can matter more than 10* (Bloomsbury, London, 1996)

Hayman, Suzie *Making the Honeymoon Last* (Hodder & Stoughton, 2000)

Inlander, Charles B. et al. *Men's Health and Wellness Encyclopaedia* (Macmillan, New York, 1998)

Korda, Michael *Man to Man: Surviving Prostate Cancer* (Warner Books, London, 1998)

Martin, Paul *The Sickening Mind: Brain, Behaviour, Immunity and Disease* (Flamingo, London, 1997)

Ornish, Dean *Love and Survival: The Scientific Basis for the Healing Power of Intimacy* (HarperCollins, New York, 1998)

Real, Terrence *I Don't Want to Talk About It: Overcoming the secret legacy of male depression* (Fireside, New York, 1998)

Warburton, Diana *A-Z of Aphrodisia* (HarperCollins, London, 1995)

Breast changes

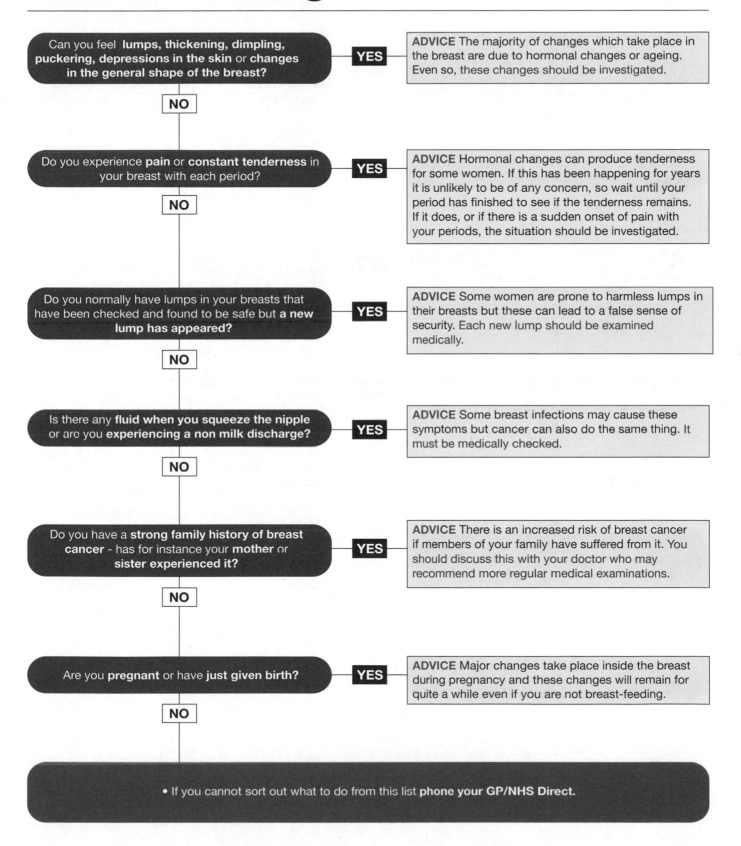

Can you feel **lumps, thickening, dimpling, puckering, depressions in the skin** or **changes in the general shape of the breast?**

YES — **ADVICE** The majority of changes which take place in the breast are due to hormonal changes or ageing. Even so, these changes should be investigated.

NO

Do you experience **pain** or **constant tenderness** in your breast with each period?

YES — **ADVICE** Hormonal changes can produce tenderness for some women. If this has been happening for years it is unlikely to be of any concern, so wait until your period has finished to see if the tenderness remains. If it does, or if there is a sudden onset of pain with your periods, the situation should be investigated.

NO

Do you normally have lumps in your breasts that have been checked and found to be safe but **a new lump has appeared?**

YES — **ADVICE** Some women are prone to harmless lumps in their breasts but these can lead to a false sense of security. Each new lump should be examined medically.

NO

Is there any **fluid when you squeeze the nipple** or are you **experiencing a non milk discharge?**

YES — **ADVICE** Some breast infections may cause these symptoms but cancer can also do the same thing. It must be medically checked.

NO

Do you have a **strong family history of breast cancer** - has for instance your **mother** or **sister** experienced it?

YES — **ADVICE** There is an increased risk of breast cancer if members of your family have suffered from it. You should discuss this with your doctor who may recommend more regular medical examinations.

NO

Are you **pregnant** or have **just given birth?**

YES — **ADVICE** Major changes take place inside the breast during pregnancy and these changes will remain for quite a while even if you are not breast-feeding.

NO

• If you cannot sort out what to do from this list **phone your GP/NHS Direct.**

Depression

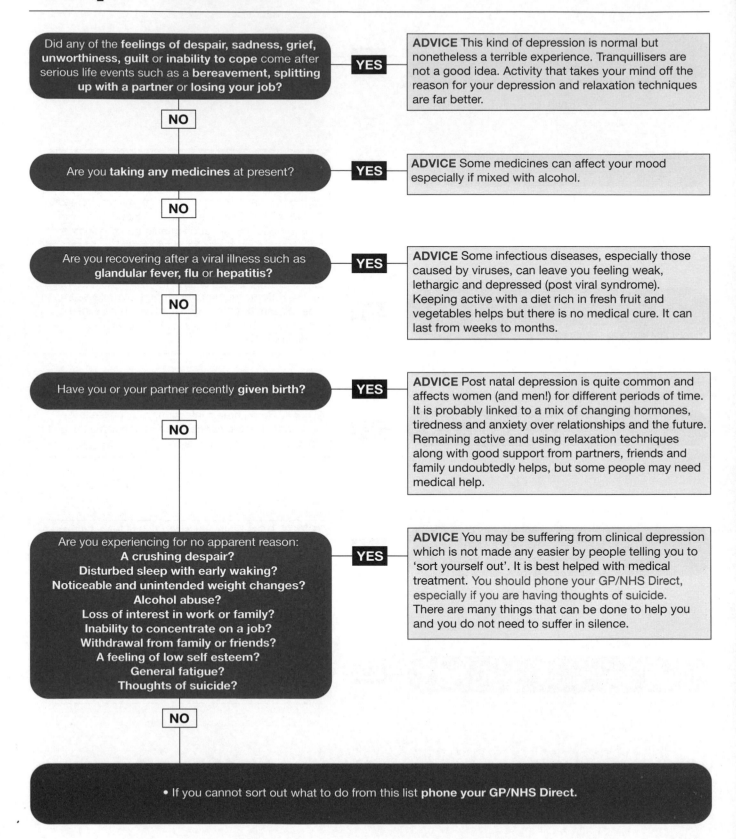

Did any of the **feelings of despair, sadness, grief, unworthiness, guilt** or **inability to cope** come after serious life events such as a **bereavement, splitting up with a partner** or **losing your job?**

YES → **ADVICE** This kind of depression is normal but nonetheless a terrible experience. Tranquillisers are not a good idea. Activity that takes your mind off the reason for your depression and relaxation techniques are far better.

NO

Are you **taking any medicines** at present?

YES → **ADVICE** Some medicines can affect your mood especially if mixed with alcohol.

NO

Are you recovering after a viral illness such as **glandular fever, flu** or **hepatitis?**

YES → **ADVICE** Some infectious diseases, especially those caused by viruses, can leave you feeling weak, lethargic and depressed (post viral syndrome). Keeping active with a diet rich in fresh fruit and vegetables helps but there is no medical cure. It can last from weeks to months.

NO

Have you or your partner recently **given birth?**

YES → **ADVICE** Post natal depression is quite common and affects women (and men!) for different periods of time. It is probably linked to a mix of changing hormones, tiredness and anxiety over relationships and the future. Remaining active and using relaxation techniques along with good support from partners, friends and family undoubtedly helps, but some people may need medical help.

NO

Are you experiencing for no apparent reason:
A crushing despair?
Disturbed sleep with early waking?
Noticeable and unintended weight changes?
Alcohol abuse?
Loss of interest in work or family?
Inability to concentrate on a job?
Withdrawal from family or friends?
A feeling of low self esteem?
General fatigue?
Thoughts of suicide?

YES → **ADVICE** You may be suffering from clinical depression which is not made any easier by people telling you to 'sort yourself out'. It is best helped with medical treatment. You should phone your GP/NHS Direct, especially if you are having thoughts of suicide. There are many things that can be done to help you and you do not need to suffer in silence.

NO

• If you cannot sort out what to do from this list **phone your GP/NHS Direct.**

Erectile dysfunction

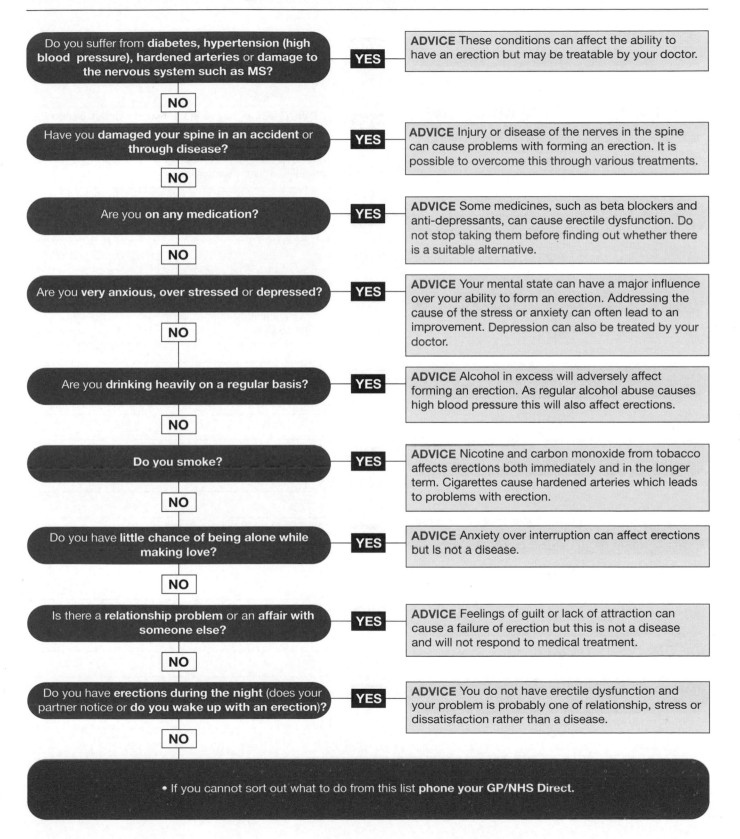

Do you suffer from **diabetes, hypertension (high blood pressure), hardened arteries** or **damage to the nervous system such as MS?** — **YES** → **ADVICE** These conditions can affect the ability to have an erection but may be treatable by your doctor.

NO

Have you **damaged your spine in an accident** or **through disease?** — **YES** → **ADVICE** Injury or disease of the nerves in the spine can cause problems with forming an erection. It is possible to overcome this through various treatments.

NO

Are you **on any medication?** — **YES** → **ADVICE** Some medicines, such as beta blockers and anti-depressants, can cause erectile dysfunction. Do not stop taking them before finding out whether there is a suitable alternative.

NO

Are you **very anxious, over stressed** or **depressed?** — **YES** → **ADVICE** Your mental state can have a major influence over your ability to form an erection. Addressing the cause of the stress or anxiety can often lead to an improvement. Depression can also be treated by your doctor.

NO

Are you **drinking heavily on a regular basis?** — **YES** → **ADVICE** Alcohol in excess will adversely affect forming an erection. As regular alcohol abuse causes high blood pressure this will also affect erections.

NO

Do you smoke? — **YES** → **ADVICE** Nicotine and carbon monoxide from tobacco affects erections both immediately and in the longer term. Cigarettes cause hardened arteries which leads to problems with erection.

NO

Do you have **little chance of being alone while making love?** — **YES** → **ADVICE** Anxiety over interruption can affect erections but Is not a disease.

NO

Is there a **relationship problem** or an **affair with someone else?** — **YES** → **ADVICE** Feelings of guilt or lack of attraction can cause a failure of erection but this is not a disease and will not respond to medical treatment.

NO

Do you have **erections during the night** (does your partner notice or **do you wake up with an erection)?** — **YES** → **ADVICE** You do not have erectile dysfunction and your problem is probably one of relationship, stress or dissatisfaction rather than a disease.

NO

• If you cannot sort out what to do from this list **phone your GP/NHS Direct.**

Irregular periods

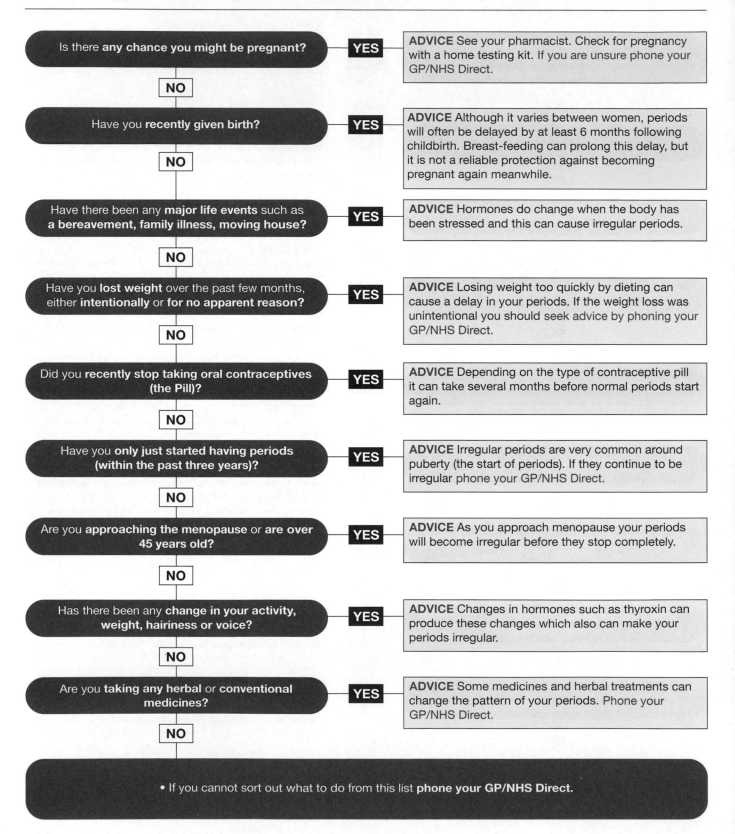

Is there **any chance you might be pregnant?** → **YES** → **ADVICE** See your pharmacist. Check for pregnancy with a home testing kit. If you are unsure phone your GP/NHS Direct.

NO

Have you **recently given birth?** → **YES** → **ADVICE** Although it varies between women, periods will often be delayed by at least 6 months following childbirth. Breast-feeding can prolong this delay, but it is not a reliable protection against becoming pregnant again meanwhile.

NO

Have there been any **major life events** such as **a bereavement, family illness, moving house?** → **YES** → **ADVICE** Hormones do change when the body has been stressed and this can cause irregular periods.

NO

Have you **lost weight** over the past few months, either **intentionally** or **for no apparent reason?** → **YES** → **ADVICE** Losing weight too quickly by dieting can cause a delay in your periods. If the weight loss was unintentional you should seek advice by phoning your GP/NHS Direct.

NO

Did you **recently stop taking oral contraceptives (the Pill)?** → **YES** → **ADVICE** Depending on the type of contraceptive pill it can take several months before normal periods start again.

NO

Have you **only just started having periods (within the past three years)?** → **YES** → **ADVICE** Irregular periods are very common around puberty (the start of periods). If they continue to be irregular phone your GP/NHS Direct.

NO

Are you **approaching the menopause or are over 45 years old?** → **YES** → **ADVICE** As you approach menopause your periods will become irregular before they stop completely.

NO

Has there been any **change in your activity, weight, hairiness or voice?** → **YES** → **ADVICE** Changes in hormones such as thyroxin can produce these changes which also can make your periods irregular.

NO

Are you **taking any herbal** or **conventional medicines?** → **YES** → **ADVICE** Some medicines and herbal treatments can change the pattern of your periods. Phone your GP/NHS Direct.

NO

• If you cannot sort out what to do from this list **phone your GP/NHS Direct.**

Tight foreskin (phimosis)

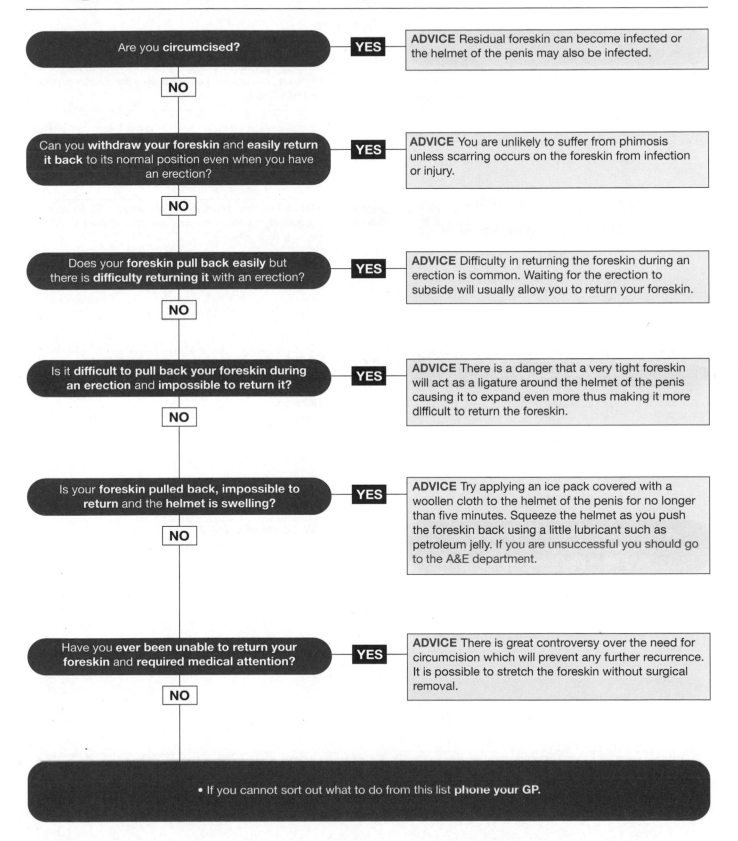

Are you **circumcised?**

YES ADVICE Residual foreskin can become infected or the helmet of the penis may also be infected.

NO

Can you **withdraw your foreskin** and **easily return it back** to its normal position even when you have an erection?

YES ADVICE You are unlikely to suffer from phimosis unless scarring occurs on the foreskin from infection or injury.

NO

Does your **foreskin pull back easily** but there is **difficulty returning it** with an erection?

YES ADVICE Difficulty in returning the foreskin during an erection is common. Waiting for the erection to subside will usually allow you to return your foreskin.

NO

Is it **difficult to pull back your foreskin during an erection** and **impossible to return it?**

YES ADVICE There is a danger that a very tight foreskin will act as a ligature around the helmet of the penis causing it to expand even more thus making it more difficult to return the foreskin.

NO

Is your **foreskin pulled back, impossible to return** and the **helmet is swelling?**

YES ADVICE Try applying an ice pack covered with a woollen cloth to the helmet of the penis for no longer than five minutes. Squeeze the helmet as you push the foreskin back using a little lubricant such as petroleum jelly. If you are unsuccessful you should go to the A&E department.

NO

Have you **ever been unable to return your foreskin** and **required medical attention?**

YES ADVICE There is great controversy over the need for circumcision which will prevent any further recurrence. It is possible to stretch the foreskin without surgical removal.

NO

• If you cannot sort out what to do from this list **phone your GP.**

Female urinary problems

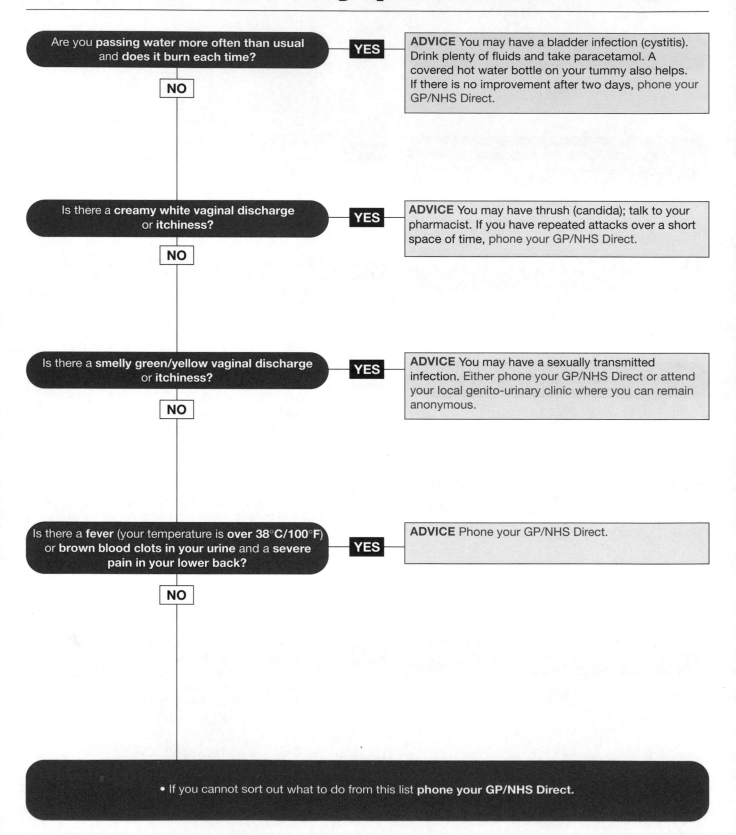

Are you **passing water more often than usual** and **does it burn each time?**

YES

ADVICE You may have a bladder infection (cystitis). Drink plenty of fluids and take paracetamol. A covered hot water bottle on your tummy also helps. If there is no improvement after two days, phone your GP/NHS Direct.

NO

Is there a **creamy white vaginal discharge** or **itchiness?**

YES

ADVICE You may have thrush (candida); talk to your pharmacist. If you have repeated attacks over a short space of time, phone your GP/NHS Direct.

NO

Is there a **smelly green/yellow vaginal discharge** or **itchiness?**

YES

ADVICE You may have a sexually transmitted infection. Either phone your GP/NHS Direct or attend your local genito-urinary clinic where you can remain anonymous.

NO

Is there a **fever** (your temperature is **over 38°C/100°F**) or **brown blood clots in your urine** and a **severe pain in your lower back?**

YES

ADVICE Phone your GP/NHS Direct.

NO

• If you cannot sort out what to do from this list **phone your GP/NHS Direct.**

Male urinary problems

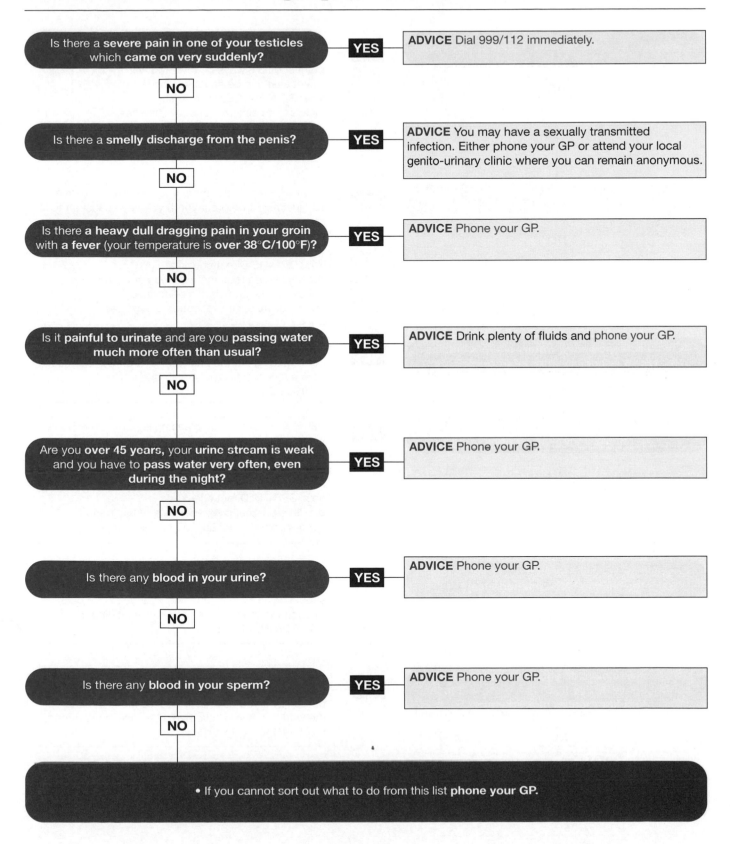

Is there a **severe pain in one of your testicles** which **came on very suddenly?** — **YES** → **ADVICE** Dial 999/112 immediately.

NO

Is there a **smelly discharge from the penis?** — **YES** → **ADVICE** You may have a sexually transmitted infection. Either phone your GP or attend your local genito-urinary clinic where you can remain anonymous.

NO

Is there **a heavy dull dragging pain in your groin** with **a fever** (your temperature is **over 38°C/100°F)?** — **YES** → **ADVICE** Phone your GP.

NO

Is it **painful to urinate** and are you **passing water much more often than usual?** — **YES** → **ADVICE** Drink plenty of fluids and phone your GP.

NO

Are you **over 45 years,** your **urine stream is weak** and you have to **pass water very often, even during the night?** — **YES** → **ADVICE** Phone your GP.

NO

Is there any **blood in your urine?** — **YES** → **ADVICE** Phone your GP.

NO

Is there any **blood in your sperm?** — **YES** → **ADVICE** Phone your GP.

NO

• If you cannot sort out what to do from this list **phone your GP.**

Vaginal bleeding

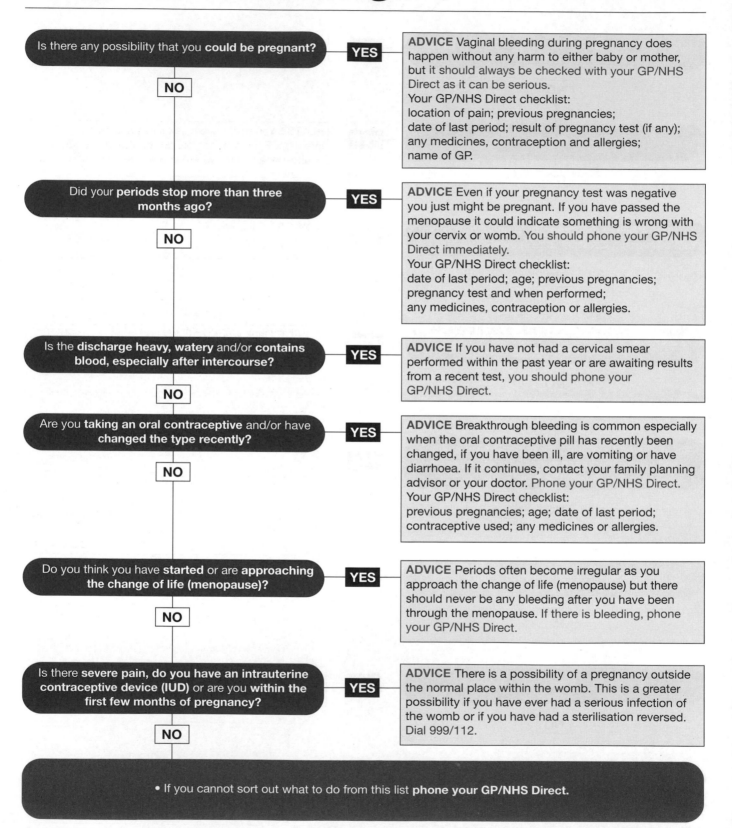

Is there any possibility that you **could be pregnant?** → **YES**

ADVICE Vaginal bleeding during pregnancy does happen without any harm to either baby or mother, but it should always be checked with your GP/NHS Direct as it can be serious.
Your GP/NHS Direct checklist:
location of pain; previous pregnancies;
date of last period; result of pregnancy test (if any);
any medicines, contraception and allergies;
name of GP.

NO

Did your **periods stop more than three months ago?** → **YES**

ADVICE Even if your pregnancy test was negative you just might be pregnant. If you have passed the menopause it could indicate something is wrong with your cervix or womb. You should phone your GP/NHS Direct immediately.
Your GP/NHS Direct checklist:
date of last period; age; previous pregnancies;
pregnancy test and when performed;
any medicines, contraception or allergies.

NO

Is the **discharge heavy, watery** and/or **contains blood, especially after intercourse?** → **YES**

ADVICE If you have not had a cervical smear performed within the past year or are awaiting results from a recent test, you should phone your GP/NHS Direct.

NO

Are you **taking an oral contraceptive** and/or have **changed the type recently?** → **YES**

ADVICE Breakthrough bleeding is common especially when the oral contraceptive pill has recently been changed, if you have been ill, are vomiting or have diarrhoea. If it continues, contact your family planning advisor or your doctor. Phone your GP/NHS Direct.
Your GP/NHS Direct checklist:
previous pregnancies; age; date of last period;
contraceptive used; any medicines or allergies.

NO

Do you think you have **started** or are **approaching the change of life (menopause)?** → **YES**

ADVICE Periods often become irregular as you approach the change of life (menopause) but there should never be any bleeding after you have been through the menopause. If there is bleeding, phone your GP/NHS Direct.

NO

Is there **severe pain, do you have an intrauterine contraceptive device (IUD)** or are you **within the first few months of pregnancy?** → **YES**

ADVICE There is a possibility of a pregnancy outside the normal place within the womb. This is a greater possibility if you have ever had a serious infection of the womb or if you have had a sterilisation reversed. Dial 999/112.

NO

• If you cannot sort out what to do from this list **phone your GP/NHS Direct.**

Dimensions and weight

1 More than half of us men are overweight – and the proportion is increasing by about one per cent a year. But it doesn't have to be like this; we don't have to resign ourselves to the slow but steady creep of so-called 'middle-age spread'.

Why bother to lose weight?

2 You'll feel better. As you're able to exert greater control over your body size and shape:

a) *Your self-esteem and self-confidence will rise.*

b) *You'll have more energy. That's because your body won't be using up so much simply carrying itself around.*

c) *Your penis could start to look longer as abdominal fat can conceal up to two inches.*

d) *Your sex drive will increase. As you lose weight, your testosterone levels will start to rise, boosting your libido and improving your fertility.*

e) *You'll snore less. Snorers are generally overweight.*

f) *You'll live longer. Being overweight is actually a bigger risk factor than smoking for heart disease. Your risk of heart disease, certain cancers, diabetes, gall bladder disease and a range of bone, joint and skin disorders will fall as you lose weight.*

The fat facts

3 Lighter men live longer on average. A man of any age who weighs 11.5 stone and is 5 feet 10 inches tall has a 30% lower risk of dying in any given year than a man of the same height who weighs 16.5 stone.

4 Non-obese men generally have healthier hearts. A man with a body mass index (BMI) of 22 or 23 is about half as likely to suffer from major coronary heart disease as a man with a BMI of over 30. He is also over eight times less likely to develop diabetes.

5 A 20% rise in body weight creates an 86% greater risk of heart disease.

6 Losing weight can lower blood pressure.

7 Obese men are more likely to develop cancer. There's strong evidence linking obesity to an increased risk of colon cancer, especially in men who are also physically inactive.

8 Being overweight increases the risk of arthritis.

Are you overweight?

9 There are three easy ways of working out whether your health could be at risk.

The waist test

10 Your circumference is a good, rough-and-ready indicator of your overall body fat level. Simply stand up and find your natural waist line (it's mid-way between your lowest rib and the top of the hip bone). Place a tape around this line and take a measurement after relaxing your abdomen by breathing out gently. If you measure 37-39.5 inches, you're technically overweight. If your waist tops 40 inches, then you're clinically obese.

The body mass index

11 There are two ways to calculate your body mass index (BMI):

a) *Using pounds and inches. Multiply your weight in pounds by 700 and divide that figure by the square of your height in inches. For example, if you're 68 inches tall and weigh 185 lb, your BMI = 185 x 700 ÷ (68 x 68 = 4624) = 28.*

b) *Using kilograms and metres. Dividing your weight by the square of your height. This means that if you're 1.78 metres tall and weigh 78kg, your BMI = 78 ÷ (1.78 x 1.78 = 3.2) = 24.4.*

12 Ideally, your score should be between 20 and 25 (in fact, a BMI of about 22 is probably best for long-term health); below 20 and you're underweight; between 25 and 30, you're overweight; and if you're above 30, you're obese. This is the standard test used to check whether your weight could cause health problems. It's not so suitable for fit men with loads of muscle, however, since they could seem overweight even though they're actually carrying very little fat.

Height / weight chart – Imperial (height in inches, weight in pounds)

Height	Underweight	Healthy weight	Overweight	Obese
63	up to 113	113 – 141	141 – 169	169 plus
64	up to115	115 – 144	144 – 173	173 plus
65	up to 121	121 – 151	151 – 182	182 plus
66	up to 124	124 – 155	155 – 186	186 plus
67	up to127	127 – 159	159 – 191	191 plus
68	up to 132	132 – 165	165 – 197	197 plus
69	up to 135	135 – 168	168 – 202	202 plus
70	up to 140	140 – 174	174 – 209	209 plus
71	up to143	143 – 178	178 – 214	214 plus
72	up to 147	147 – 184	184 – 221	221 plus
74	up to 155	155 – 194	194 – 233	233 plus
75	up to 159	159 – 199	199 – 238	238 plus

Height / weight chart – metric (height in metres, weight in kilograms)

Height	Underweight	Healthy weight	Overweight	Obese
1.60	up to 51	51 – 64	64 – 77	77 plus
1.63	up to 52	52 – 65	65 – 79	79 plus
1.65	up to 55	55 – 69	69 – 83	83 plus
1.68	up to 56	56 – 70	70 – 84	84 plus
1.70	up to 58	58 – 72	72 – 87	87 plus
1.73	up to 60	60 – 75	75 – 89	89 plus
1.75	up to 61	61 – 76	76 – 92	92 plus
1.78	up to 64	64 – 79	79 – 95	95 plus
1.80	up to 65	65 – 81	81 – 97	97 plus
1.83	up to 67	67 – 84	84 – 100	100 plus
1.88	up to 70	70 – 88	88 – 106	106 plus
1.91	up to 72	72 – 90	90 – 108	108 plus

The waist : hip ratio

13 Measure your waist and hips. (It doesn't matter whether you do this in centimetres or inches.) Measure the circumference of your waist as described in the waist test; your hips should be measured at their widest part.

14 Divide your waist measurement by your hip measurement to get a ratio. For example, if your waist is 90cm and your hips 105cm, the ratio is 0.86. If your ratio is greater than 0.95, you need to lose some weight. This is a particularly useful test because it assesses your fat distribution and calculates whether you have too much around your abdomen.

What car?

A few suggestions from our resident experts. Feel free to add your own...

Caterham 7

• This is one of the harder efforts but a standing canine position is possible over the roll bar.

Escort Mexico with roll cage (or any other car with a cage)

• The tubes give something useful to hold onto to prevent exhaustion in the legs and can also be used for those handcuff moments but you do have to remember to mind your head.

Land Rover Discovery

• If this was a bed it would be a king size. Plenty of room means virtually anything's possible. A lot of glass though which can lead to embarrassment!

Mini

• One of the favourites I'm sure. Early models virtually impossible, but by C reg the seats could tilt and so some positions possible, best I think is man on the back seat, legs apart and female in the front leaning over giving head. This enables the handbrake to be brought into play as well!

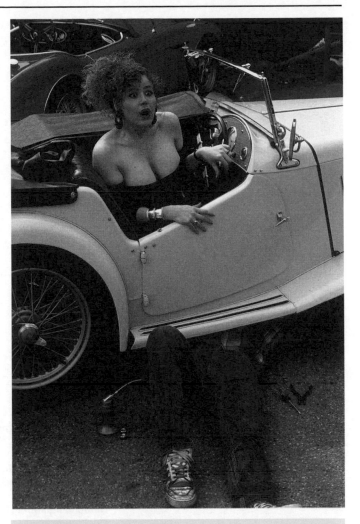

Ever tried it in a mini? My advice is to make sure you don't inadvertently switch on the radio with your foot, as the faint sound of someone talking, apparently just a few feet away, can repeatedly disturb even the most avid of young lovers, especially when in a dark lonely Scottish car park. It happened to a friend of mine...

Reliant Robin

• Don't laugh, there's lots of room and the gear lever is only held in by a spring clip. Mind it doesn't tip over, though.

Renault Kangoo

• Lower the back seats to form a flat surface, except for the side on which you will rest both your heads. Both partners use the erect seat for their heads and curl up in an S position – with the man at the back of the female. The penis will enter the vagina from the back, thus stimulating the woman's clitoris and penetrating at the same time. She cuddles up to the man as close as she can in a foetal position – as the kangaroo offspring is in the pouch. A fun position which will get you hopping with pleasure.

Triumph Spitfire

• The idle is always so rough, it adds a new dimension to having sex on the bonnet...

Index

Credits

Cover models	Nina, Jodie Frapple
Cover photography	Simon Dodd
Editor	Ian Barnes
Editorial director	Matthew Minter
Page build	James Robertson
Photo credits	Page 2•24 © Pictorial Press; page REF•15 © REX by David McEnery / Rex Features; page REF•19 © Touchstone Films
Production control	Kevin Heals
Tales and tips	Ian Barnes, Martine Bradshaw, Ian Campbell, Jeremy Churchill, John Fowler, Michael Hamilton, Annette Haynes, J. Haynes, Kevin Heals, Bob Jex, Chris Wall, Bow Watkinson, Alan White
Technical illustrations	Roger Healing and Mark Stevens

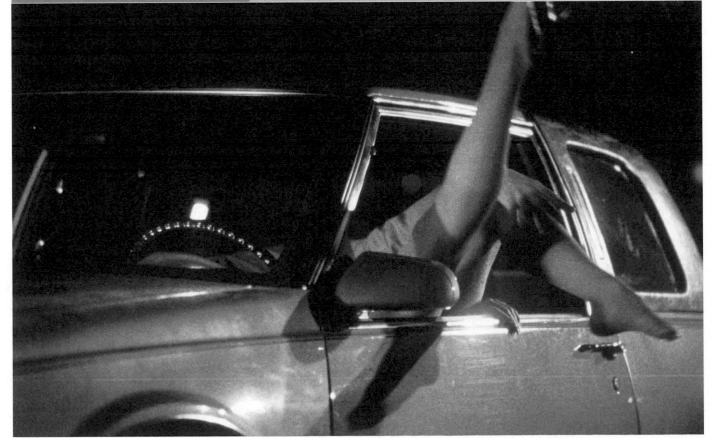

Oops a daisy!

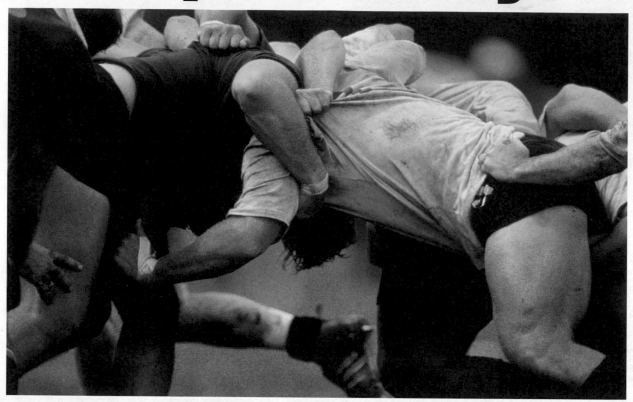

Though it's sometimes hard to believe, even the lumpiest forward started out life as a tiny, vulnerable baby. Luckily there's plenty of information on sports injuries in the **Haynes Man Manual** - and a lot more besides. Check your own tackle, give our tricks of the trade a try, and kick your health problems into touch.

Also available in a Junior version.

For every copy of the Man Manual sold, 50p is donated to the Men's Health Forum for their work in tackling cancer. For every copy of the Baby Manual sold, 50p is donated to the Great Ormond Street Children's Hospital Charity.

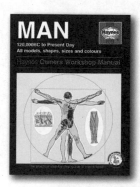
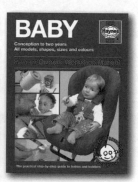

Both these manuals are available from branches of Halfords, WH Smith, Waterstone's, Ottakar's and most other high street bookshops, price **£12.99** each. They can also be purchased direct from Haynes by calling 01963 442030 or by visiting www.haynes.co.uk

Haynes Publishing, Sparkford, Yeovil, Somerset BA22 7JJ